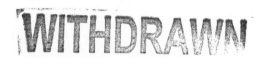

The Anti-Aging Solution

5 Simple Steps to Looking and Feeling Young

Vincent Giampapa, M.D.

Ronald Pero, Ph.D.

Marcia Zimmerman, CN

Foreword by Nicholas Perricone, M.D.

WILEY

John Wiley & Sons, Inc.

Published by John Wiley & Sons, Inc., Hoboken, New Jersey
Published simultaneously in Canada

Design and production by Navta Associates, Inc.

For general information about our other products and services, please contact our Customer Care Department within the United States at (800) 762-2974, outside the United States at (317) 572-3993 or fax (317) 572-4002.

Wiley also publishes its books in a variety of electronic formats. Some content that appears in print may not be available in electronic books. For more information about Wiley products, visit our web site at www.wiley.com.

ISBN 0-471-47932-2

Printed in the United States of America

10 9 8 7 6 5 4 3 2 1

CONTENTS

FOREWORD

In my first book, *The Wrinkle Cure,* I wrote the following words: "Aging is optional. We don't have to age like our parents. We can hold on to our vitality and look well into our later years." Although this has been a long cherished conviction of mine, little did I know that it was destined to become a rallying cry of a new generation of adults—a generation of highly educated and motivated men and women who are committed to optimizing and maintaining their health, beauty, and well-being for as long as humanly possible.

This phenomenon is not just limited to baby boomers but appears to have struck a chord with people in their twenties and thirties as well. I find this tremendously inspiring, because if we are going to keep this great country vital, our citizens need to be strong, healthy, and as self-sufficient as possible. Programs such as I outlined in *The Perricone Prescription* and that Dr. Giampapa and his coauthors have so brilliantly and lucidly put forth in *The Anti-Aging Solution: 5 Simple Steps to Looking and Feeling Young* are the tools we need to ensure that this can happen. When we lower our stress, make the right food choices, take targeted nutritional supplements, and follow a moderate yet effective fitness program, we are well on our way to achieving the dream of a long, healthy, and active life into our final decades.

In addition to their own cutting-edge research, Dr. Giampapa and his coauthors have gathered the proven research of many scientists to present the Anti-Aging Solution 5-Step Plan. By understanding the scientific basis of how and why we age, we can finally begin to halt and slow the process.

> —Nicholas Perricone, M.D.
> Adjunct Professor of Medicine
> Michigan State University College of Human Medicine
> Best-selling author of *The Wrinkle Cure*
> and *The Perricone Prescription*

ACKNOWLEDGMENTS

The Anti-Aging Solution would never have emerged without a hard-working team of people. Special thanks go to our agents, Jenny Bent and Harvey Klinger in New York, and to our editor at John Wiley and Sons, Tom Miller, and his assistant Kellam Ayres. They have made extraordinary efforts to get the cutting-edge information contained in this book into the hands of readers in record time.

Anti-Aging Medicine with a focus on DNA repair is on the cusp of twenty-first-century wellness. Many scientists and physicians have contributed to this information and we acknowledge their contributions. The research team in the Department of Cell and Molecular Biology, University of Lund, Lund, Sweden, includes: Yezhou Sheng, M.D., D.M.Sc., Anders R. Olsson, Ph.D., Jianyi Hua, M.D., and Carl Bryngelsson, B.Sc. Physicians who practice anti-aging medicine and who have collaborated with Dr. Giampapa include: Eric Braverman, Ward Dean, Bob Goldman, Thierry Hertoge, Dharma Khalsa, Ron Klatz, Steve Novell, Chong Park, and Steven Sinatra.

Introduction

Science headlines announce daily some new discovery made using information gleaned from the Human Genome Project. We read about finding a new disease gene or a key protein linked to some condition. While this information is interesting, it holds little practical application to our daily lives. Development of drugs designed to alter genes and the way they work is still in the future and is fraught with uncertainties.

This book is also about genes. However, the information contained here *is* of practical application, is available *now,* is scientifically validated, and has been proven clinically safe and effective at the Giampapa Institute in Montclair, New Jersey, as well as at other clinical institutions worldwide. For the first time, you will be able to take charge of your health by applying The Anti-Aging Solution 5-Step Plan to your personal Aging Equation. This book uses mind/body therapies to alter your aging process and improve your quality of life. It is based on over 30 years of solid scientific research and has been fine-tuned through 20 years of clinical practice. You will meet the patients of Dr. Giampapa who have enjoyed years of looking and feeling young simply by following his 5-Step Plan. Dr. Pero has collaborated with Dr. Giampapa in developing the first anti-aging program centered on DNA repair.

There has been major interest in the topic of aging ever since humans began surviving long enough to contemplate their future. Hundreds of years ago, Ponce de León is said to have found Florida while searching for the fountain of youth. Yet scientists weren't particularly interested in the aging process until the 1960s, when staggering health care costs for the elderly began driving research dollars into anti-aging medicine. The percentage of the elderly making up the world's population continues to increase.

The World Health Organization estimates that by 2005 there will be 800 million people over age 65, accounting for one in ten individuals. Between 1990 and 2000, the number of people 65 or older in the United States alone increased by 12 percent from 31.3 million to 35 million. That number is expected to increase by 34 percent over the next 20 years to 46.9 million.

Clearly, the demand for anti-aging therapies will increase. The American Academy of Anti-Aging Medicine (A4M) was founded in 1993 to meet the needs of a population demanding a new approach in medical care—one designed to stall the aging process and extend a healthy life span. Vincent Giampapa, M.D., is one of six founding physicians of A4M and a former president of the association. Dr. Giampapa has also chaired the board that certifies physicians in the anti-aging specialty. Today there are over 2,000 physician members of A4M.

These physicians are on the cutting edge of medicine and many practice complementary medicine. This discipline uses conventional medicine when appropriate but prefers the more benign therapy of diet and supplements. Complementary medicine is becoming increasingly validated as more research uncovers how nutrients affect aging.

What these physicians have discovered in the practice of anti-aging medicine is now available to you. Armed with this information, you can take charge of your life and extend your healthy and productive years.

A 60-year old psychologist from New York is an outstanding example of the success of the 5-Step Plan laid out in this book. Mary came to Dr. Giampapa 18 years ago complaining of fatigue, insomnia, weakness, inability to concentrate, poor memory, dry skin, and thinning hair—all typical signs of aging with no identifiable cause. Dr. Giampapa did a comprehensive workup on Mary that included an extensive lifestyle and health history interview plus the Giampapa anti-aging panel of laboratory tests. He was particularly interested in her nutrition, fitness, and stress-reducing practices. Dr. Giampapa calls this evaluation *factoring the Aging Equation,* and it's different for every patient. Laboratory tests showed low levels of key vitamins and minerals, hormone imbalances, specifically high cortisol/low thyroid, and inability to correctly utilize dietary carbohydrates. Mary's prescription called for dramatic dietary change, stress-reducing techniques, a daily exercise plan, and a topical cream designed to balance hormones, repair DNA, and rejuvenate her skin.

Today, Mary is a small dynamo (5'3" and 112 pounds) regularly working 12- to 13-hour days to maintain a busy counseling practice. Her mind is sharp and she has no trouble staying focused. She requires less sleep with improved sleep quality. Her low-carbohydrate diet emphasizing lots of antioxidant-rich vegetables, a little fruit, and high-quality protein has resolved her low blood sugar problems. Her skin is smooth and radiant and she has thicker hair.

You will meet other patients of Dr. Giampapa and learn how the 5-Step Plan has improved their lives. They are living testimony that growing older doesn't necessarily equate with aging. All of us grow older, but aging is a choice!

The new millennium is sweeping in unprecedented scientific and medical advances in genomic research. The remarkable unraveling of the human genome, unquestionably the most significant scientific discovery of the last half century, is changing the practice of anti-aging medicine. While the Human Genome Project offers the promise of a new approach to aging, it also opens the door to taking greater personal responsibility for your own aging.

There is a clear cause and effect between aging conditions, your diet, and lifestyle. Consequently, you can apply much of this new information to take charge of your own aging process. You don't have to give in to achy joints, sagging skin, and fatigue. Make a few simple changes in your life and reap incredible benefits that you can see and feel in just a few days.

The Anti-Aging Solution differs from any other anti-aging book in that it attacks aging at its genetic roots with a comprehensive plan. The book shows how to improve the quality and function of the genetic material that fills each of your 100 trillion cells. It tells you about a natural compound extracted from the herb *Uncaria tomentosa* that has emerged from solid scientific research and been proven to ratchet up genetic repair systems within each cell.

The book also tells you how to get the most anti-aging benefits from foods you may already have in your kitchen simply by combining them for color and adding antioxidant and enzyme-activating spices.

We show you that sugar is poison for your skin, leads to storage of fat around your middle, and raises levels of the aging hormone cortisol. Your mirror gives testimony to external aging effects, but what you don't see are the internal effects that come from the same aging processes. We show you how to rejuvenate your skin and body by altering genetic function while improving internal cellular function. Modifying simple daily activities will help you achieve fitness goals, sculpt a more youthful body contour, improve memory, increase energy levels, and relieve the severity of age-related conditions.

The beauty and strength of this genetic approach to anti-aging is that nothing has been left out when considering the root causes of age-associated disease. A solution to the maze of interacting aging processes is reduced into the Anti-Aging Solution 5-Step Plan:

Step 1: Reduce your stress.
Step 2: Nourish your genes.
Step 3: Exercise your genes.
Step 4: Supplement your genes.
Step 5: Make over your skin and body.

Genetic damage is the ultimate reason why we succumb to various age-related conditions. *Reversing this damage is the only way to reverse aging.*

Let's begin by describing the indicators that make up the Aging Equation.

PART ONE

Your Aging Equation

I don't want to achieve immortality through my work; I want to achieve it through not dying.

—*Woody Allen*

CHAPTER 1

Finding Your Personal Aging Equation

Old age is far more than white hair, wrinkles, the feeling that it's too late and the game finished, that the stage belongs to the rising generations. The true evil is not the weakening of the body, but the indifference of the soul.

—*Andre Maurois*

One day it suddenly hits us—we're growing older! It's usually around our thirtieth birthday that we begin to realize we're not kids anymore, and although we may feel just as youthful in spirit, our body is beginning to show signs of aging. We start thinking about how to stay young as long as possible, perhaps becoming more diet conscious, taking up regular exercise, and adding dietary supplements as extra health insurance. Grant's story is pretty typical of many people. He wanted to counter the effects of aging but was surprised that it entailed a 5-step process:

I read an article entitled "Grow Young with HGH" and saw Dr. Giampapa's name in the bibliography, and I decided to go and visit him because I live near his office. I didn't have any specific complaints—just wanted to stay young and healthy as long as possible.

The office visit wasn't your typical one. We discussed my situation at great length and I was impressed with what he had to say.

7

He then set me up for complete blood work. Really complete! Based on the information he got back, he set me up with three high-protein gourmet meals a day, daily exercise, a supplement program, and DHEA cream. That was 3 years ago, and since that time Dr. G has periodically checked my blood work and made adjustments in my supplement program.

I feel great, but I felt great when I went to Dr. G's. But by comparison, I believe I have more energy now, which I thought was impossible. I believe my body has more muscle, less fat (wasn't fat to begin with). Waist has decreased from 33–34 back to 32–33. But I do feel younger and I definitely don't feel any older. I'm 55 and I feel 25.

Dr. G's regimen has also helped me with stress control and anger management through the use of tryptophan and other supplements.

Grant has stuck with Dr. Giampapa's program despite his misgivings. He is enthusiastic about how effective the 5-Step Plan has been and the surprising benefits such as a positive mental outlook.

Are you aging and willing to undertake the necessary steps to stay young and healthy as long as possible? The Anti-Aging Solution will show you how to do just that. Let's begin by checking aging signs that you may be experiencing.

Aging has an unpleasant connotation. Few of us are willing to admit we are aging. It often takes a wake-up call to interest us in taking better care of ourselves. Doctors recognize these wake-up calls as *clinical endpoints,* a term that reinforces a decidedly negative connotation. Yet these are precisely the kind of indicators that the 5-Step Plan addresses and that you can control. We're going to call them *aging indicators.* The following list has some that you may have personally encountered. However, you probably haven't associated them with aging, especially since many can occur in children and young adults as well, based on their genetic inheritance. Some of the most common aging signs include

overweight	lagging energy	sleep problems
chronic pain	chronic sinusitis	skin sensitivity/rash
constant stress	forgetfulness	difficulty concentrating
poor memory	reduced mobility	allergies, chronic
digestive complaints	variable appetite	rhinitis

decreased immunity	hormone	frequent infections
skin lesions/	imbalances	nervousness, fatigue
sun spots	gum disease	sore joints
lagging libido	digestive problems	irritable bowel
		syndrome

The intensity of these conditions is determined by your genetic inheritance but is also seriously influenced by your environment. You may have struggled with some of these conditions for years, with symptoms worsening at certain times of the year or alleviated by a change of lifestyle or environment. You can expect childhood conditions to intensify as you get older, with related symptoms appearing. For example, you may have had seasonal hay fever as a child, but as you grow older the attacks most likely will intensify. They are precipitated by an increasing number of environmental triggers, and you may have added other allergic symptoms such as skin allergies. That's why it's important that you identify your aging indicators and use this book to overcome them.

Allergies involve inflammation that often leads to more serious conditions such as asthma and cardiovascular disease. In fact, inflammation is considered one of the hallmarks of disease. Here are a few simple tests for you to try that will show you why you need to follow the Anti-Aging Solution 5-Step Plan.

How Quickly Are You Aging?

Skin Elasticity

Loss of skin elasticity starts to be significant in your forties (around age 45) and is the direct result of the underlying deterioration of proteins that make up skin tissue—namely collagen and elastin. This loss of skin tone appears as wrinkles on your face and loose skin around your jowls and neck. Pinch the skin on the back of your hand between your thumb and forefinger for 5 seconds. Release it, and time how long it takes the skin to flatten out completely. This is an indicator of your biological or real age. It may or may not correspond to your chronological age.

0–1 second = 20–30 years of age
2–5 seconds = 40–50 years of age
10–55 seconds = 60–70 years of age

By enhancing DNA repair, skin fibroblasts produce healthier, more youthful cells.

Reaction Time

The "falling ruler" tool is a measurement of your reaction time that falls off sharply with aging. Use an 18-inch wooden ruler and have someone hold the 1-inch end of the ruler at the top. Using your dominant hand, leave a 3½-inch space between your thumb and forefinger. The other person should let go of the ruler without warning and you should try to grab it as quickly as possible between your fingers before it hits the floor. Note the inch mark where you grabbed the ruler. Do this three times and average the results.

> 12 inches = 20–30 years of age
> 8 inches = 40–50 years of age
> 5 inches = 60–70 years of age

You can improve your reaction time by strengthening your small muscle groups, which is part of our fitness makeover.

Static Balance

This test determines how long you can stand on one leg with your eyes closed before losing your balance. Stand on a hard surface (not a rug) with both feet together. You should be barefoot or wearing a low-heeled shoe. Try this exercise first with your eyes open, and if it's fairly easy, try closing your eyes. Lift your foot—left foot if right handed; right foot if left handed—about 6 inches off the ground, bending your knee about 45 degrees. Stand on your other foot without moving or jiggling it. Have someone time how long you can do this without either opening your eyes or moving your foot to avoid falling. Do this three times, average, and record.

> 28 seconds = 20–30 years of age
> 18 seconds = 40–50 years of age
> 4 seconds = 60–70 years of age

It's amazing how many 20-year-olds can't do this exercise, and you may have to start with your eyes open and touching the wall for stability. Loss of balance is an aging condition that sneaks up on us and seriously reduces our quality of life. It can also lead to accidents. You can dramatically increase your ability to balance, thereby reducing your tendency for injury, just by following our anti-aging exercises.

Visual Accommodation

With age, the lens of your eye becomes progressively less elastic, resulting in nearsightedness. The following is not a totally accurate test; however, it will give you some idea of the effect of age on your vision. Hold a newspaper in front of you while you are not wearing prescription lenses. Slowly bring the newspaper to your eyes until the regular-size letters start to blur. Have someone measure the distance from your eyes to the newspaper. Record.

> 4.5 inches = 20–30 years of age
> 12 inches = 40–50 years of age
> 39 inches = 50–60 years of age

Are your arms getting shorter? People who have always been nearsighted may ace this one! The supplements we recommend may actually improve your vision by reducing free radical damage to your eyes and improving the ability to focus.

Body Composition

This measurement will provide you with a good idea of your fat to lean muscle mass ratio or percent of body fat. Obtain a skin-fold caliper from your local health food shop or fitness center. Calipers are simple to use once you get the hang of them. Make two skin-fold measurements in each of the specified locations, and record the percentage of fat indicated on the calipers. Repeat three times. The measurements should not vary more than 1 percent. Women use the skin fold on the top of the hip bone and on the back of the upper arm. Men use the skin fold on the front of the thigh and on the back of the upper arm. The caliper records skin fold in millimeters (mm). You will have to use a conversion table provided with the caliper to change millimeters into percent body fat. Ideal body fat content for men is 15 to 17 percent; for women it is 18 to 22 percent. Our menu and fitness exercises will tone and reshape your body to achieve a better fat to lean muscle mass ratio. Calipers have about a 5 percent error factor. Many fitness clubs are now offering hydrostatic body fat or bioimpedance analysis for a more accurate measurement.

Body Mass Index

Body mass index (BMI) measures your ratio of lean body mass to fat. It has some limitations in that the calculation for very muscular individuals may indicate being overweight. However, combined with the caliper reading, BMI is a useful tool and quite accurate for most of us. Measure your height and weight using the same equipment each time. Divide your weight in pounds by the square of your height in inches, then multiply by 703 to calculate your BMI.

> 20–25 BMI = ideal
> 26–30 BMI = overweight
> 31–34 BMI = obese
> 35 or higher BMI = extremely (morbidly) obese

Waist to Hip Ratio

Body mass index is a good overall measure of the lean muscle to fat ratio, but very muscular people should remember that muscle is much heavier than fat. A good alternative is the waist to hip ratio (WHR), which is your waist size divided by your girth at the broadest part of your buttocks. The waist measurement for both genders is taken just above the hip bones and over the navel. Women are accustomed to measuring their waist for clothing at the narrowest part of their torso, but this doesn't apply for WHR. Lower numbers—0.85 or below—indicate that you have relatively little fat over your abdomen and are at lower risk for heart attack and stroke.

The emphasis in the menu and fitness exercises is on body composition more than weight. This is how the eating and hormone balancing parts of the Anti-Aging Plan differ from weight-loss plans. You will improve your body composition without dieting.

Skin elasticity, reaction time, static balance, visual accommodation, body composition, BMI, and WHR are in fact a panel of simple noninvasive *objective measures* that can be used every day in your home to help you evaluate the effectiveness of the Anti-Aging Plan. You do not have to rely only on your *subjective measures* of feeling better or worse but can objectively judge your anti-aging progress through utilization of the panel of aging procedures that measure early clinical manifestation of aging.

You should now fill out the Subjective Questionnaire in appendix B. As you proceed through the 5-Step Plan, you will be checking your symptom improvement. We also suggest you utilize the home tests we provide in the appendix. These will give you an objective assessment measure of your progress with the Anti-Aging Solution 5-Step Plan.

Mind/Body Connection in Aging

Aging has been defined as a decline in an individual's ability to adapt to environmental, psychological, and physiological stress that leads to the development of flaws within the immune system. Such flaws can be the direct result of oxidative stress and DNA damage. They can also be an indirect assault on genes from an infection or a stressful lifestyle because these events increase oxidative burden.

Aging is characterized by a decline in the body's immune responsiveness, with an increasing appearance of disease conditions such as cancer, atherosclerosis, high blood pressure, diabetes, and arthritis. There are two types of immune cells: B cells and T cells. While B cells produce antibodies, T cells regulate the activities of other white blood cells, which in turn send signals through the immune, nervous, and glandular systems.

As we age, the immune function of these cells declines, particularly that of T cells. The ratio between various kinds of T cells is altered, with an overproduction of pro-inflammatory cells and a decrease in anti-inflammatory cells. T cells become less aggressive in attacking invading organisms and increasingly lax in regulating B cells and other white blood cells. As a result, the tendency for self-destruction of one's tissues (autoimmunity) increases. Scientists estimate that 10 to 15 percent of seemingly healthy older individuals have increased blood levels of antibodies against their own tissues.

The thymus gland produces generic (undifferentiated) stem cells that can be programmed into different kinds of immune cells. The thymus gland is most active when we are children, and it actively communicates with the hypothalamus and pituitary glands in the brain. As we age, the thymus shrinks in size with decreased production of stem cells.

It is widely accepted within the scientific community that most aging conditions have a basis in immune dysfunction. Moreover, there is now clear-cut evidence that information is constantly being exchanged between the central nervous system and the immune system. Thus how you think and feel has a direct impact on your immune response. A new branch of medicine called psychoneuroimmunology has emerged since the mid-1970s. It is the study of interactions between behavior, the nervous system, and the immune system. A substantial body of evidence has revealed that the brain has a major influence on the immune/inflammatory response by communicating with hormones and peripheral nerves.

The brain sends messages using special chemicals known as *cytokines,* which are messenger proteins produced by immune cells to communicate with one another. Cytokines also converse with the nervous system, providing a system of checks and balances between the brain and the immune system. Cytokines act on surface receptors in brain cells, which activate nerve cells throughout the body. There are many different kinds of cytokines; TNFα is the primary one that you will encounter as you read this book.

Stress and Immune Response

Immune system mediators such as cytokines are released in response to stress. Stressful events may stem from physical injury or infection, or they can have a psychological origin. Regardless of the source, the mind/body response involves the same set of mediators.

Injury or infection triggers inflammation to stem the flow of microbes and promote healing. Associated "illness behaviors" such as sleep disturbances, lack of appetite, apathy, and sluggishness are familiar to most of us. These result from the nervous system response to illness. After a few days, the infection resolves and you begin to feel normal. However, inflammation can persist well past the stage of infection, with psychological stress being a major cause of its persistence. Enduring psychological or physical stressors—poor diet is one—affect the central nervous system and induce an unremitting adrenaline rush. This is nature's way of helping us cope. Adrenaline and the hormone cortisol activate the fight-or-flight response with which most of us are all too familiar. Today's fast-paced lifestyle causes surges in cortisol and adrenaline that keep us in an inappropriate state of readiness to combat an unseen enemy.

Digestive disturbances are one of the first complaints we have when we go through periods of intense stress. Energy is being diverted from the gastrointestinal tract to energize muscles, increase blood flow, and heighten alertness to enable escape from pending danger. Infection or trauma causes a drop in appetite, whereas psychological stress will likely increase snacking and possibly lead to binge eating. In addition to the effect on appetite and digestion, stress hormones alter cellular function and cause imbalances among other hormones including insulin and the sex hormones. Unremitting psychological stress leads to a cycle in which cytokines promote inflammation and accelerate aging by increasing damage to cells and genes.

Stress and Inflammation

A recent study found that biomedical students taking final exams had increased levels of inflammation. Moreover, those students who were the most stressed had the highest levels of inflammatory mediators. It's not unusual for students to succumb to postexam illness. Many of us have a similar response after a stressful period such as after a hectic holiday season, work project, or personal matter. Stressful situations occur throughout life, but our ability to cope lessens as we age. Controlling stress is the first step in the Anti-Aging Solution, and it's the topic of chapter 3.

Inflammation is now considered by leading heart experts to be a primary cause of atherosclerosis or arterial blockage. This information is changing the way physicians assess your risk of heart disease. Buildup of plaque narrows the interior of arteries, blocking blood flow, increasing the pressure on arterial walls, and leading to blood clot formation. Experts have maintained for a number of years that the kind of plaque that builds up is especially notable. Inflammation generates a very unstable plaque that is soft and squishy. As the plaque "ripens," it ruptures and spews forth its inflammatory products, including one called *C-reactive protein.*

C-Reactive Protein: Something Worse Than Cholesterol?

C-reactive protein (CRP) indicates chronic inflammation. Initially it is produced to fight infection, help clear away dead bacteria, and promote healing. As long as inflammation persists, blood levels of CRP remain high. If this condition is prolonged, it will likely play a role in atherosclerosis. CRP levels are one of the best tools for identifying future risk of cardiovascular disease.

The process of inflammation and arterial scarring goes on silently for years before a stroke or heart attack. Now that doctors know CRP levels are elevated whenever inflammation persists, they can predict risk of cardiovascular events years before disease symptoms appear. Thus, routine screening for blood levels of CRP is being advocated by many experts, among them Drs. Zebrack and Anderson from the University of Utah School of Medicine. They suggest that early testing for CRP is not only a useful indicator for future risk of cardiovascular disease but a better predictor than other commonly used tests such as total cholesterol and triglycerides.

Paul Ridker, M.D., of Boston's Brigham and Women's Hospital, conducted two large studies that confirm the usefulness of CRP testing. The first study involved 1,086 male physicians and the second 27,939 healthy nurses. Male physicians having the highest levels of CRP, many of them smokers, had three times the risk for heart attack and twice the risk for stroke than those with the lowest levels. However, smoking wasn't the only cause of chronic inflammation, since many physicians with high CRP levels had never smoked. Moreover, the strong association of CRP with future heart attack was not affected by other known risk factors such as body mass index, diabetes, hypertension, high triglycerides, high total cholesterol, low HDL (good) cholesterol, and family history. Nevertheless, men having both high cholesterol and CRP may have up to nine times the risk of heart attack.

In the women's study the relative risk of a first cardiovascular event was more strongly associated with high levels of CRP than high LDL (bad) cholesterol. Surprisingly, half of the women with high CRP had normal cholesterol levels. Yet having high LDL cholesterol in addition to high CRP didn't seem to increase risk. This finding helps provide new insight as to why only half of women having a first heart attack have high levels of LDL cholesterol. Chronic inflammation may be an even better predictor of cardiovascular disease in women than in men.

CRP levels are an especially good indicator of risk of future heart attack for younger individuals for whom dietary and lifestyle change might have the greatest impact in altering the course of disease. CRP is easily measured, inexpensive, and widely praised as the best indicator of future cardiovascular events, particularly for women.

Infection as a Basis for Cardiovascular Disease

Low-grade infection plays a significant role in cardiovascular disease as we have seen, but where does the infection come from? Several scientific investigators have found that prior infection with *Chlamydia pneumoniae, Helicobacter pylori,* herpes simplex virus, *Streptococcus,* or cytomegalovirus (CMV) led to chronic inflammation with resulting high levels of CRP. It has been recognized for many years that rheumatic fever, an acute streptococcal infection, can cause damage to heart valves. A recent study has shown that streptococcal infections weaken heart muscle as well. *Chlamydia* appears to be most connected with cardiovascular disease, although *H. pylori* and CMV are also implicated.

Chlamydiae are a family of parasites that infect the respiratory membranes including those of the eyes and lungs. They are transmitted by contact between contaminated fingers and eyes but also from the moist cough or saliva of another person. *Chlamydia* infections can cause one type of pneumonia. If left untreated or not killed by antibiotics, *Chlamydia* can persist for many years.

Helicobacter pylori causes gastritis and peptic ulcers. It is also a risk factor for stomach cancer. *H. pylori* attaches to the stomach lining, causing persistent inflammation that leads to tissue damage and loss of the protective mucous lining of the stomach. Stomach acid then burns the unprotected stomach wall, causing ulceration. Antibiotics are also used to treat *H. pylori,* but it can be difficult to eradicate.

Herpes simplex and cytomegalovirus are related viruses that cause oral and genital warts (herpes) and immune suppression of T cells. Both can be transmitted by saliva or sexual contact. CMV can pass into the fetus from the placenta or infect the newborn from breast-feeding.

Streptococcal bacteria are normally found on skin surfaces and cause problems only when they gain entry into the body. They are a common threat to patients in weakened conditions such as nursing mothers, newborns, and those hospitalized or with a serious illness. Acute infections are treated with antibiotics but can damage internal organs if left untreated.

Doctors in Salt Lake City, Utah, found *Chlamydia* infection was associated not only with arterial plaque but also with angina, heart attack, and stroke. They found patients with arterial narrowing not only had antibodies against CMV but also had high levels of CRP. The Utah doctors found that high homocysteine, another factor associated with cardiovascular disease, is particularly risky when paired with high CRP. Patients with the highest levels of homocysteine were nearly 16 percent more likely to die of cardiovascular disease. The risk was even higher if homocysteine and CRP were both high. Besides the infectious factors discussed here, there are other microbes that play a role in cardiovascular disease.

Austrian doctors found that microbes causing chronic respiratory, urinary tract, dental, and other infections amplified the risk of developing arterial plaque and also led to autoimmune conditions such as rheumatoid arthritis. Moreover, they suggested that chronic respiratory infections, which are common among smokers, might underlie the high rates of atherogenesis—that is, abnormal fatty deposits in the arteries—found in this group.

Using This Information

If you have had a serious infection or have a chronic inflammatory condition such as allergies, rashes, asthma, chronic sinusitis, arthritis, or autoimmune conditions, you should consider having your CRP level tested. If your level is high, indicating chronic infection, the responsible microbe can be identified by laboratory analysis, which detects antibodies that your immune system has produced to fight the microbe. Diagnostic laboratories that do these tests are listed in the resources section of this book.

Dental health is also important in preventing cardiovascular disease. Several important studies have shown the connection between periodontitis, a common form of chronic infection, and cardiovascular disease. You will want to concentrate on foods that reduce inflammation and add supplements to fight infection. As for damage to your genes, the tests we suggest in appendix A will show you what effect chronic inflammation has had. You can then use the suggested measures that might include bumping up DNA repair and/or additional antioxidant supplements or topical hormones that are suggested in chapters 6 and 7. If the infection is ongoing, you should consult your physician.

It is possible for you to control much of your own aging. Oxidative stress and its consequences are the predominant cause of aging. Damage to DNA, reduced DNA repair capability, altered genetic expression, visible signs of aging, and chronic inflammation are all critical factors in considering how to live a longer, healthier life. From the evidence presented, we can now show how the Anti-Aging Solution 5-Step Plan will help you.

Let's move on to how aging occurs.

CHAPTER 2

How Aging Occurs

Age does not depend upon years, but upon temperament and health. Some men are born old, and some never grow so.
—*Tyrone Edwards*

Our biological clock starts ticking when we're born. Yet until age 30 or so, we grow better as we grow older. We overcome various childhood diseases, passing through the pains of adolescence into adulthood. Most of us—but not all—are well beyond age 30 before we begin to experience signs of aging such as skin wrinkling, hair graying, various aches and pains, low energy, fatigue, reduced stress adaptation, lowered immune response, decreased muscle mass, hearing loss, and vision problems. These are generally accepted as part of growing older and we look to our genetic heritage to check how we'll age.

Aging and Your Genes

At the heart of the Human Genome Project is the mapping of deoxyribonucleic acid or DNA, the material that makes up our genes. Genes contain explicit codes that direct all vital cellular functions, and it's on this level that the Anti-Aging Solution works. Although you can't do much about the genes you inherit—body composition, hair and eye color—you can change the way your genes express themselves by exercising the 5 steps in our plan. To better understand this plan, you need to know a little more about DNA.

DNA, Genes, and Chromosomes

All organisms contain DNA, which carries the code for survival of the species. Amazingly, only four letters—A, G, T, and C—make up this code, and human DNA contains roughly 3.2 billion A, G, T, and Cs; the letters are shorthand for names of the bases that make up DNA— adenine, guanosine, thymine, and cytosine. The code is spelled out with repeating units containing these four letters. The four letters connect in only one way—A always pairing with T, and G with C—thus ensuring that the code is copied exactly every time DNA reproduces itself. The assembled DNA molecule resembles a long spiraling staircase with the paired letters A-T and G-C forming its steps. A specific sequence of these paired letters represents a gene.

DNA is too small to see with the highest resolution microscope. If we could see it, the DNA in each cell would be 5 feet in length but only 50 millionths of an inch wide. Nature manages this unwieldy molecule by tightly coiling it around special proteins called histones, and this is how DNA is stored in the nucleus.

The dense coiled strands of DNA containing the genetic code are called *chromatin*. Students of biology can view these strands under a light microscope as they uncoil in preparation for cellular division. Two identical chromatin strands make up each of the 46 chromosomes in your cells. The chromosomes are paired into 22 identical sets plus a set of sex chromosomes that are paired in females (XX) but not in males (XY).

Amazingly, 99.9 percent of DNA found in the human body is identical in all people. It's the remaining 0.1 percent that holds the key to understanding disease. To date, there have been 923 of these "disease genes" identified. Thirty-one percent of disease genes encode enzymes. We'll soon explain the importance of enzymes, especially as they relate to aging and aging conditions. Now let's move on to an explanation of how small genetic modifications supply your personal identity.

Genetic Variations

The Human Genome Project has revealed a bumper crop of human genetic variations called single-nucleotide polymorphisms, or SNPs, pronounced "snips." These are the smallest possible genetic changes that can occur in DNA, and they help give us our individual blueprint for life. Unlike DNA damage that leads to aging, SNPs are an important evolutionary characteristic that enables us to adapt to an ever-changing environment. Nearly 1.5 million SNPs have already been identified, and they are providing a powerful tool in studying human diseases and human history.

SNPs account for individual differences in drug metabolism and response. Among the proteins encoded by SNPs are a group of liver enzymes that are responsible for metabolizing and clearing drugs from the system. Individual differences in these enzymes explain why some people have adverse reactions to medications at normal doses, whereas others experience adverse reactions at higher or lower doses. *Designer therapeutics* is a whole new field that takes into account individual reactions to a specific therapy.

SNPs might also be used to predict individual needs for specific supplements or foods. For example, some individuals do not metabolize vitamin B_6 (pyridoxine) properly. They might need higher doses of pyridoxine or respond better to the more bioavailable coenzyme form called pyridoxal-5-phosphate (P_5P). Others may need higher doses of specific antioxidants. There are no scientific data available yet to validate this clinical approach to individualizing treatment with diet and supplements based on gene snips, but it is the future of personalized anti-aging medicine.

Remarkable new advances in stem cell research, proteomics (gene-expressed protein patterns), gene splicing, and drug therapy aimed at genes are already changing the practice of medicine in the twenty-first century. Molecular medicine offers exciting new horizons for altering the course of aging, and an even greater potential benefit might be gleaned by applying genomic information to nutritional anti-aging medicine.

Genetic Control of Aging

Scientists have been deciphering aging codes on genes and have now identified at least eight genes that can influence longevity. The goal of most anti-aging research involves manipulating these genes either by physical or chemical means to extend life span and overcome various aging conditions. While your genetic makeup helps determine how you age, many scientists believe that longevity has more to do with how you live than with your genetic makeup. How you live is up to you, and it's the basis for the suggestions in this book.

How Genes Work

Genes are located in the command center of every cell—the nucleus. To the amazement of scientists who were expecting to find over 100,000 human genes, the Human Genome Project revealed that only 30,000 genes control the extremely complex human being. That's only about one-third more than the nematode, a little worm that eats the roots of vegetables in your garden.

Moreover, about 90 percent of those 30,000 genes were thought to have no apparent purpose or function. At first, genetic experts called them "junk DNA." In 2000–2003, scientists discovered that the so-called junk DNA appears to contain specific "how to" instructions for proteins to express themselves. A more appropriate name, introns, has now been given to these bits of DNA. The new discovery helps explain how so few genes can direct the incredibly complex processes in the human body.

Your marvelous genes direct thousands of different metabolic reactions because of tiny variations in the proteins they encode. Scientists estimate that 4,096 human genes have these small variations, each gene giving rise to 576 different proteins that each bear a slightly different amino acid sequence. Amino acids are the basic units that are strung together to build proteins. It's the vast number of variant proteins that allow us to function as humans and adapt to our ever-changing environment. If we change our environment for the better, we can change our genetic expression and how our proteins work. This is the basis of the Anti-Aging Solution.

Genetic Reproduction

Your genes reproduce (replicate) themselves, with the typical cell dividing approximately 70 times before dying. The duplication process begins as the paired strands of DNA uncoil from around histone proteins and start unzipping up the middle. The open-ended letters (bases) are now joined to their appropriate base partner: A to T and G to C selected from a pool of letters in the nucleus. As the letters are properly hooked up, the entire strand of DNA zips back up, forming two exact copies of the original.

The extraordinary fidelity with which DNA replication occurs billions of times over a lifetime depends on certain proteins. In test tube experiments, if DNA is denied the help of these proteins, it inserts the wrong letter approximately once in every 100 attempts. Yet, when combined with the appropriate proteins, only one mistake occurs in every 10 million insertions.

As you age, the duplication process becomes less than perfect, with nicks, strand breaks, and fragmentation of DNA occurring. As a consequence, genetic expression is altered, which dramatically changes the face of what it means to grow older. The essence of the Anti-Aging Solution is repairing these flaws in DNA.

Protein Chaperones and Protein Folding

Newly minted proteins including the all-important enzymes are long, flat ribbons with no particular shape for interacting with target molecules. They must be folded into an organized ball-like structure with their reactive sites tucked among the folds.

Smaller proteins appropriately named *chaperones* carefully fold their larger unwieldy cousins into tight packages with their reactive sites tucked safely inside. Other chaperones guide the folded proteins to the correct location in the cell. Nobel Laureate Günter Blobel has compared this process to affixing a zip code to the protein so that it arrives at its assigned location in the cell. Misfolded proteins are implicated in at least twenty diseases including Alzheimer's, Parkinson's, and Creutzfeldt-Jakob disease, the human variation of mad-cow disease.

Genetic Switches

Fine-tuning of genetic expression occurs throughout life as genes that are not needed are switched off while those that must be active are switched on. Switching genes off and on is a clever way for the body to conserve effort and preserve genetic stability. Early in life, growth-directing genes are switched on. As you get older, growth genes are silenced and those that repair your body are switched on.

Genetic switches are actually methyl (CH_3) groups attached to the cytosine base in DNA. These tiny "wings" modify genetic architecture, thus changing genetic expression and enzyme activity. Approximately 4 percent of cytosine bases in DNA are normally methylated or switched off at any given time. The rest are switched on (unmethylated). Strict control over genetic switching gives the body stability and preserves good health and longevity.

As you age, greater numbers of genes are switched off, dramatically altering cellular chemistry and contributing to the development of cancer and certain nerve and brain disorders. Lung and colorectal cancers have been linked to errors in gene switching. Fortunately, good nutrition helps safeguard proper gene switching and can help overcome incorrect switching.

Genetic Expression

The genetic code is transferred when a single strand of DNA links up with the transcription molecule ribonucleic acid or RNA. The letter bases in RNA must line up with those in DNA so that the genetic sequence is transferred. RNA now bearing the genetic code for building proteins transcribes the code to enzymes that assemble amino acids in a specified order for building the desired protein. These proteins then express genetic instructions with a dizzying array of variants, as already described, which modify their function. Scientists call this *post-transcription modification.* Many of the proteins encoded by DNA are the all-important metabolic enzymes; they are the biological catalysts for thousands of different cellular activities. The ability of these enzymes to adapt is how your body maintains its homeostasis.

Why Enzymes Are Important

There are approximately one billion protein molecules in each cell and approximately twelve percent are enzymes. The Human Genome Project has now catalogued 3,870 metabolic enzymes, each controlling a specific event. Nearly all require a vitamin coenzyme and many also need a mineral cofactor to activate them. Enzymes are extremely sensitive to deficiencies of vitamins and minerals, with metabolism slowing down dramatically during periods of nutrient deficit. When these cofactoring nutrients are restored, enzyme function resumes and health improves. Most of us think nutrient deficiency means eating too little food, and of course starvation will deprive us of nutrients. However, few of those living in developed countries are in danger of starvation. Instead, most people eat too much food that has been stripped of vitamins and minerals. They eat enough calories to pack on pounds yet leave their cells starved for the necessary vitamins and minerals. They are malnourished.

Nutrition and Enzyme Function

Nutritional deficiencies occur long before they're evident in standard blood tests or with symptoms recognized by most physicians. Measuring intracellular levels of vitamins, minerals, and fatty acids and assessing overall antioxidant status can detect nutrient deficits. However, this type of assessment is still not widely employed even though there are good laboratory tests available. There are also tests that measure DNA damage and identify its enhanced repair. These tests can give you a jump-start on controlling your own aging. We tell you how and where to get them in appendix A and in the resources section.

Why Do We Age?

Free radicals are the primary cause of aging. They are highly charged atoms, molecules, or compounds that are missing one electron, making them unstable. Electrons possess tremendous energy, and this energy drives atoms to bond and form molecules. Electrons normally pair up, but if enough external energy is supplied—for example, ultraviolet light—one of the paired electrons may be knocked off. An atom with a single electron seeks a second one, which it steals from a neighboring atom that must now gain its own electron. The process of electron swiping disrupts normal cellular processes, wreaking havoc. Electrons are easier to steal from some molecules with DNA, fatty acids and proteins being prime targets.

At least 300 modern theories of aging have been proposed. The most accepted one is the free radical theory of aging. In 1956, Denham Harman, M.D., at the time a professor at the University of California, Berkeley, proposed that free radical reactions, regardless of how they are initiated, are responsible for the progressive deterioration of biological systems seen over a lifetime. The free radical theory has matured over the years as details of how free radicals cause deterioration and illness have been revealed.

Leonard Hayflick, Ph.D., a well-known anti-aging researcher also from UC Berkeley, has stated, "Aging is an accumulation of random damage to the building blocks of life—especially to DNA, certain proteins, carbohydrates, and lipids (fats)—that begins early in life and eventually exceeds the body's self-repair capabilities."

Fatty Acid Damage and Its Consequences

Polyunsaturated fatty acids (PUFAs) are a fertile source of electrons because they contain several exposed electron pairs. It's easy for free radicals to sneak in and swipe one of these electrons, which sets off a cascade of destructive activity. As one fatty acid is robbed of its electrons, it scrambles to replace them with a widespread negative impact on cellular function. While PUFAs are an energy source for cells, they fill a more important role as integral components of membranes. They contribute to membrane stability, cell communication, hormone and neurotransmitter function, growth and differentiation. Transport of nutrients, oxygen, and other important chemicals across the membrane is blocked and numerous cellular functions are altered when membrane fats are attacked.

Sources of Free Radicals

Free radicals come from the environment, smoking, and various toxins we ingest, including medications. However, most are produced within your own cells as a normal by-product of converting food into energy. Mitochondria are the power plants of the cell that produce energy (ATP) from glucose and oxygen. ATP is the energy-rich molecule that drives metabolism, and it is continually recycled in order to supply the energy needs of your body. These energy-producing reactions aren't 100 percent efficient, and some oxygen molecules become free radicals as mitochondrial enzymes recycle ATP. A single ATP molecule must be recycled within a mitochondrion approximately 1,000 times per day for the body to maintain its energy supply. There are thousands of ATP molecules in every mitochondrion, and some cells have hundreds of mitochondria.

It's been estimated that about 10 percent of the air we breathe every day is turned into free radicals by mitochondrial enzymes. Anti-aging experts maintain that damage to mitochondrial DNA is particularly insidious because enzymes throughout the body depend on energy. Bruce Ames, Ph.D., professor of biochemistry and molecular biology at the University of California, Berkeley, and one of the most cited scientists in the world, has calculated that the human cell is buffeted by 10,000 free radical hits each day. What happens to your genes as a result of this bombardment?

Free Radicals Damage Your Genes

Free radicals can induce strand breaks or scramble the bases in DNA, causing the wrong letters to be inserted. In addition to direct hits on DNA, free radicals also activate a protein known as nuclear transcription factor kappa B, or NF-κB. Many agents including viral infections, oxidants, and antibodies activate this factor. Free radical activation of NF-κB leads to an increase in inflammatory and immune responses. Chief among them is the cytokine TNFα. These two factors interact, egging each other on in promoting inflammation.

NF-κB attaches to genes that promote inflammatory conditions such as allergies, asthma, rheumatoid arthritis, inflammatory bowel disease, and psoriasis. It also activates genes that promote tumor growth and blocks other genes that increase tumor cell destruction. Obviously, NF-κB promotes aging through these destructive activities.

Agents such as antioxidants that block NF-κB have the ability to alter the aging process. Chief among these is a newly discovered class of compounds known as carboxy alkyl esters (CAEs) that are found in a proprietary water-soluble extract of cat's claw *(Uncaria tomentosa)*. This extract is an essential tool for attacking aging at its genetic roots.

Free Radicals and Genetic Expression

Damaged genes cannot pass on accurate instructions for the production of enzymes and other proteins. Consequently, a series of events that cause aging and age-related conditions is set in motion.

DNA Damage, Health Consequences

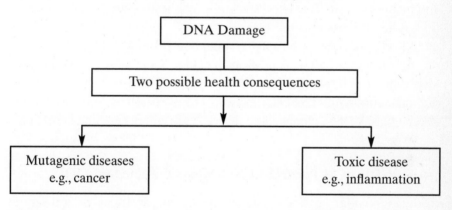

How Does Your Body Cope with Free Radical Damage?

Nature has provided an internal antioxidant system to deactivate free radicals before they can harm you. The system is headquartered in the liver, but cells also have their own antioxidant system. This system becomes less efficient as with age, and mounting oxidative stress produces damage to genes. Your body depends on a generous supply of antioxidants from the food you eat. A diet rich in fruit, vegetables, herbs, and spices provides the backup for your internal antioxidant system. The menu makeover in chapter 4 will show you which foods you should eat to provide a powerhouse of antioxidants. In addition, supplements including a wide range of antioxidants are suggested in chapter 6.

Apoptosis: A Two-Edged Sword in Aging

The cellular life span consists of approximately seventy divisions. When they have outlived their usefulness, cells accept a signal from DNA that it's time to self-destruct. The process of cellular suicide is called *apoptosis,* and it's one of the most important events in preserving your youth and vigor. There is an important connection between apoptosis and inflammation.

The inflammatory agent TNFα triggers the signal that leads to apoptosis. Yet TNFα can no longer promote apoptosis when exposed to oxidative stress, radiation, certain chemotherapeutic drugs, or activated NF-κB. Tumor destruction is quickly negated when TNFα activates NF-κB, which then sticks to DNA and turns off apoptosis. These conditions dampened scientific hope that TNFα would increase apoptosis in cancer cells when it was discovered that it does just the opposite when goaded by NF-κB. In her wisdom, nature designed this system of checks and balances to prevent excessive apoptosis that might lead to destruction of healthy tissues.

NF-κB generates a series of events that promote aging. Being very sensitive to oxidative stress, it begins blocking apoptosis even without the involvement of TNFα. In fact, NF-κB causes TNFα to increase inflammation, depress immune cell function, and increase free radicals. NF-κB also increases DNA damage and dramatically alters genetic expression.

Why You Need a Range of Antioxidants

Reducing oxidative stress has been the major focus of anti-aging research, and the antioxidant supplements we recommend are based on this research. Dr. Ames and his colleagues have recently published breakthrough research on the previously unrecognized power of alpha-lipoic acid and acetyl-L-carnitine in reducing oxidative stress. Moreover, these antioxidants are active both topically and internally, which means they can be applied in creams, gels, or taken as capsules or tablets.

Another esteemed UC Berkeley scientist, Lester Packer, Ph.D., was the first to describe how antioxidants work together in quenching free radicals. All must be present to achieve efficient free radical scavenging, since they relieve one another of free radical burden. Vitamin E, vitamin C, lipoic acid, coenzyme Q_{10}, nicotinic acid, and glutathione neutralize free radicals by different methods, and they complement one another's efforts.

Random oxidative hits to your genes can impair cellular, tissue, and organ function and increase vulnerability to diseases such as Alzheimer's, heart disease, stroke, and cancer. Genetic damage also may increase inflammation, loss of muscle tissue and bone mass, cause a decline in reaction time, impair hearing and vision, and reduce skin elasticity.

Enhancing Genetic Repair

Nature, ever protective of your genes, provides repair enzymes that remove damaged sections of DNA and replace them with the correct sequence of letters. It's a remarkable system, first involving a set of enzymes that recognizes the specific kind of damage that's been done. A second set of enzymes moves in and cuts out the damaged section of DNA. Then a third set of enzymes puts in a replacement piece, followed by a fourth set that glues it in place and seals the seams. A final step disposes of the damaged segment.

Remarkable as this repair kit is, damage accumulates faster than it can be repaired, causing mistakes in protein and enzyme synthesis that lead to errors in metabolism. The first sign is lack of energy, followed by visible signs of aging. Aging conditions such as cancer, diabetes, stroke, Parkinson's disease, general inflammation, and tumor growth can all be traced to genetic damage. Fortunately, there is a way you can enhance DNA repair. This is breakthrough scientific evidence that is presented for the first time in this book.

CAE extract, or Uña de Gato, has been an important medicine among Peruvian natives for hundreds of years. Uña de Gato is considered sacred among the Campa Indians of Peru. They use it to treat many conditions including inflammation, infections, and cancer. It is also used to ease birthing and improve immune response in both the new mother and her child.

Ron Pero, Ph.D., one of this book's authors, carefully duplicated the CAE tea extraction methods used by the Peruvian shamans in preparing their medicine. The extract was named C-Med for Campa Medicine and 100 for 100 percent bioavailability, a unique characteristic of this proprietary extract. Dr. Pero then isolated an entirely new class of actives from this Cat's Claw extract. These are the *carboxy alkyl esters* or CAEs. Working from his lab in the Molecular Biology Department at Lund University in Lund, Sweden, Dr. Pero's team explored how CAEs work on the molecular level. The traditional use of CAE suggested the extract would reduce inflammation and boost immune response. Dr. Pero and his colleagues proved through many studies that it did indeed have these effects. They also showed exactly how it works by inhibiting NF-κB and boosting immune cell activity.

Much to everyone's amazement, CAEs were also found to stimulate natural DNA repair enzymes. CAEs are the only natural substance known to do this. Moreover, Dr. Pero and his team found that pairing the extract with the B vitamin nicotinamide, zinc, and natural carotenes increases its effectiveness because these other nutrients are the cofactors for DNA repair enzymes.

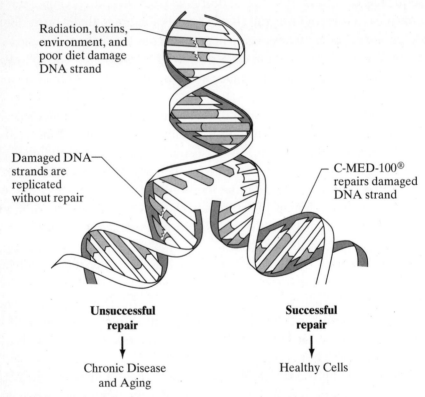

Radiation, toxins, environment, and poor diet damage DNA strand

Damaged DNA strands are replicated without repair

C-MED-100® repairs damaged DNA strand

Unsuccessful repair

↓

Chronic Disease and Aging

Successful repair

↓

Healthy Cells

Reining in Runaway Inflammation

Hormone imbalances, stress, and poor nutrition have a devastating effect on your immune system. Eliminating foods that trigger inflammation, such as sugar, alcohol, caffeine, and in some individuals, members of the nightshade family (potatoes, tomatoes, peppers), can control it. CAEs block inflammation by preventing NF-κB from sticking to DNA and blocking TNFα, while increasing tumor-killing apoptosis. As we have seen, antioxidant-rich foods and supplements help block free radicals.

The Anti-Aging Solution provides 5 steps that attack aging at its genetic roots by preventing free radical damage to DNA, enhancing its repair, and reining in runaway inflammation. It's the only anti-aging plan that does this. Moreover, the 5-Step Plan overcomes oxidative damage to the other important building blocks of life proteins, carbohydrates, and fats. It restores youthful cell function.

We are now ready to begin the 5-Step Plan that will change your life.

PART TWO

The Anti-Aging Solution 5-Step Plan

Growing old is no more than a bad habit which a busy man has no time to form.

—*Andre Maurois*

5 Easy Steps to Looking and Feeling Young

Five easy steps to solve the Anti-Aging Equation must be practiced daily. You may already be doing some of these things, but putting them all together into a cohesive plan and sticking with it is what's important. These five steps are so vital for controlling your own aging that you should commit them to memory and think about them frequently throughout the day in order.

1. Reduce your stress.
2. Nourish your genes.
3. Exercise your genes.
4. Supplement your genes.
5. Make over your skin and body.

We will explain each of these steps, then show you how they fit into a daily schedule. You can't change your nature or genetic inheritance, but you can nurture your genes to slow aging and prevent aging conditions. This is the essence of the 5-Step Plan. Begin your day with stress-reduction techniques. Follow with the other elements in the day in order.

CHAPTER 3

Step 1: Reduce Your Stress

Every stress leaves an indelible scar, and the organism pays for its survival after a stressful situation by becoming a little older.

—*Hans Selye, M.D.*

Bill's experience with Dr. Giampapa's 5-Step Plan is inspiring because he has been working on stress reduction through positive affirmations and imagery. He has also effectively embraced the other 4 steps in the plan over the past 3 months.

At 52, my hair is almost entirely gray with a receding hairline and little hair remaining down the center of my scalp. Before starting the 5-Step Plan in mid-June 2003, I weighed 193 pounds and my weight was slowly inching up. Exercise was erratic, possibly two times a week but not every week. One of my major concerns was high cholesterol, which was always above 250 and sometimes reached 270. Yet in my opinion my general health was good, having not missed a day of work due to illness in more than 2 years.

A convergence occurred when I started to take Dr. Giampapa's multiple vitamin and mineral formula with DNA repair. Summer finally arrived and I started to swim regularly around noon and on weekends in the community pool. The pool is near the office. I began listening to a tape series called *Success Through a Positive Mental Attitude* that features content from W. Clement Stone and Napoleon Hill (listening to motivation tapes is a key part of how I spend time in the car). I started to practice PMA [positive mental attitude] and created a personal affirmation that I work to say several times a day, especially while I'm driving to work. My affirmation is "I'm going forth with a happy song in my heart. I'm fearing not and sending forth love. I'm seizing the day to be confident, make sales, and produce results."

After a few weeks on the 5-Step Plan, I realized many subtle changes in strength and endurance, energy and focus level, as well as general well-being. While doing laps in the pool, I realized that I was able to swim at a moderate speed for much longer distances. The extra distance energized me to swim longer and farther. While on vacation in Canada during August, I swam in a freshwater lake and laps were 100 to 150 yards in length. I would swim for 25 to 30 minutes each day. I always walked out of the lake refreshed, energized, and not at all fatigued.

I also noticed that some hair on my head was starting to grow back. While I'll never have a full head of hair, some of the wide-open spaces on my scalp were filling in. My hair has a different texture, finer and less coarse. It is still gray and even white in some places.

While my diet has not changed dramatically, I have avoided eating empty calorie foods that I often consumed in the office or while grazing around the kitchen after work. My standard breakfast is a piece of seven-grain toast with jam and a cup of coffee around 5 A.M. Before leaving for work, I eat a bowl of fresh blueberries, grapes, chopped green apple, and other fruits with plain yogurt and some "Good Friends" cereal from Kashi. And then I take my morning dose of supplements.

This small meal keeps me going, and the dense nutrition in the supplements keeps me satisfied through the morning and into the early afternoon. Through the morning I drink seltzer or cool water from the water cooler. At lunch I usually have a sandwich and a Coke, which is a habit that I have been unsuccessful in breaking. I'm still consuming too much sugar.

After work, I arrive home with an anxiety- or stress-related need to graze on nuts and other stuff. I have switched to non-alcoholic beer instead of drinking red wine. One glass in the evening would lead to another, and I usually felt groggy and sleepy soon after the evening meal. An energy falloff would occur around 9 P.M. as my mind and body said let's lie down on the bed for a few minutes. This was a deadly pleasure, since even a 10-minute rest could quickly extend for several hours.

Then I would miss putting my children to sleep, lose the time to talk with my wife, and the evening was wasted. Dozing off at 9 P.M. would also lead to getting up at midnight, 1 or 2 A.M., and then wandering around the house awake. This late-night wakefulness would last at least an hour.

Since beginning the 5-Step Plan, increasing my exercise, reducing evening alcohol, and eating a high-protein dinner instead of grazing, the 9 P.M. slump is less pronounced.

Another simple affirmation keeps me out of bed in the mid-evening. I have picked up another affirmation from W. Clement Stone's *Positive Mental Attitude* philosophy. Stone says the best way to beat procrastination is with the simple statement "Do It Now." While lying on my bed in the early evening, Stone's "Do It Now" concept comes into my mind and I realize there are dinner dishes to be dealt with, school lunches to be made, and probably writing to do. In fact, this description was started at 11 P.M. because Stone's "Do It Now" message came to mind and so did the deadline.

Close to 90 days have passed since I began the 5-Step Plan. The first few weeks on the program I often skipped taking the supplement. Or, I'd take the supplement in the A.M. and not after dinner. Lately, however, as I began to notice improvement in my well-being, I've been taking the supplement twice a day as recommended. I have even started sharing the supplements with my wife.

What has the 5-Step Plan wrought for me? Without making an attempt to lose weight, dramatically change my diet (except I did add the morning bowl of fruit), or reduce caloric intake, my weight is now 183. This is my lowest weight in 20 years. The supplement, coupled with regular swimming (at least 20 minutes three times a week), has given my body more tone than anytime in 3 to 5 years.

My energy is up and so is my focus level. I believe that I'm getting more done and have a more positive can-do attitude toward work and the job. Daily affirmations based on PMA also help.

Dr. Giampapa's program has been very successful—it is helping me look good and feel good—even at 52. The supplements, linked with my PMA efforts, increased exercise, some changes in diet, and a desire to control or reduce my feelings of fear and anxiety, are all paying off. My cholesterol levels are down to normal and I'm looking forward to reduced allergic response as pollen season begins.

Bill's story is ideal for those of you beginning the 5-Step Plan. He has been on the program a very short time and didn't seriously undertake all 5 steps until he began to experience benefits from the few steps he had taken. His case illustrates how making even small adjustments in your diet and exercise can bring a new sense of well-being, energy, and health. As you begin to enjoy these benefits, you will be motivated to more fully embrace all 5 steps completely. The sooner you start, the more benefits you will see. And as you'll discover in the stories of others who think they are at optimum levels of energy and health, you can always benefit from the 5-Step Plan.

What Is Stress?

Stress is a normal part of life, and a certain amount is essential for survival. It allows us to respond appropriately to approaching danger or mount a defense against bacteria or viruses. A stressor can be any situation perceived as dangerous. An imagined threat or recall of a dangerous event provokes a stress response containing all the same elements as acute stress from trauma or infection. Illustrating this point, researchers at the National Institutes of Health have found a connection between depression in adults and traumas experienced in early childhood.

The primary source of stress in modern society is time urgency from an overcrowded schedule and constant stimuli and interruptions of thoughts. While multitasking we are denied the opportunity to be in the present moment, which leads to subtle but chronic changes in hormone levels, primarily cortisol.

We are also frequently exposed to rudeness, anger, anxiety, emotional upheaval, restlessness, psychological trauma, noise, crowding, isolation, hunger, danger, and infection. Real danger can come from something as routine as commuting to work and exposure to infections from those who surround us. Most of us are aware of these daily stressors, but we are less attuned to environmental stressors.

Our modern world exposes us to radiation from electromagnetic fields, surgical devices, radiological sources (X-rays), and toxic elements coming from water, food, air, household cleaners, exhaust fumes, pesticides, and sprays. Electromagnetic stressors are some of the most frequently encountered, coming from hair dryers, cell phones, cordless phones, electric blankets, and wireless communication devices. Computer monitors emit magnetic radiation from the back, and you should sit at least 3 feet from them.

Regular cell phone use may be very hazardous. A recent study by Leif Salford, M.D., of the University of Lund, Sweden, published in *Environmental Health Perspectives,* found that adolescent rats exposed (2 hours/day for 50 days) to a device emitting one-sixth the radiation of a digital cell phone experienced 2 percent brain cell death or cells in the process of dying. Cell phones are ubiquitous in modern society because they offer us a way to keep in close contact with colleagues and family members. Dr. Salford suggests keeping calls short or using a hands-free device to reduce radiation exposure.

Modern life with its unremitting psychological stress imposes an artificial fight-or-flight response. Finnish researchers recently published a 30-year study that followed 812 men and women who worked for a company in the metal industry. The scientists found that those who had the most job-related stress were over twice as likely to die of a heart attack as those in low-stress jobs. Those who felt undervalued for their contribution (low salary, lack of social approval, limited job opportunities) were two and a half times more likely to have a fatal heart attack.

While both a high-stress job and being undervalued increased risk of death from heart attack, an interesting difference in coping mechanisms emerged from these two groups of workers. Those who had stressful jobs had high cholesterol while those who had low job satisfaction gained more weight. Both of these conditions stem from elevated cortisol. However, in the first case it caused metabolic imbalance while in the second it caused insulin imbalance and possibly brain chemical disturbances that led to overeating.

What Does Stress Do to Your Cells?

Your body contains trillions of cells, each a microcosm of molecules vibrating with a specific frequency of energy. They buzz, they bump into one another, and they interact, exchanging energy as they do so and driving cellular metabolism. When you are healthy, the energy transfer is smooth and harmonious. Your whole body resonates with the dynamic flow of energy known as *vitality* or *life force.*

The flow of life's energy has been recognized for at least 7,000 years. The ancient Chinese called it *chi* or *qi,* pronounced chee, while the Hindus called it *prana.* More recently, Sigmund Freud called it *libido* and Henri Bergson referred to it as *élan vitale.* Most of us think our life force is confined to the energy within, but traditionally it has been recognized that we interact with our external environment and the energy sources outside our own body. Consequently, we can draw energy and vitality from our environment or shut it out. It's our choice that we exercise every day.

Regardless of what life's energy has been called, ill health and low energy have traditionally been viewed as unbalanced energy within the internal and external environment of the body. Healing has been focused on removing blockages to the flow of energy. How does energy transfer occur on the cellular level and what effect does stress have on it?

Membranes and Receptors

In chapter 2, we talked about how free radicals attack the oily, flexible membranes that cover the cell and its internal structures. Now, we'll tell you why this flexibility is vital to maintaining health and how the membranes function. Embedded between the membrane fatty acids are proteins that function as communication devices between cells. Just as the molecules within your cells vibrate with energy, so do the membrane's embedded proteins.

Candace Pert, Ph.D., a Georgetown University scientist who was one of the first to characterize receptor function, describes it this way. "Flexible receptor molecules respond to energy and chemical cues by vibrating. They wiggle, shimmy, and even hum as they bend and change from one shape to another, often moving back and forth between two or three favored shapes, or conformations."

We talked about protein folding and how function depends on what goes on at the reactive sites tucked within the folds. Indeed, the active sites on DNA repair enzymes are tucked within such folds. Now we can take this illustration a step further by showing that proteins actually wiggle about in order to expose reactive sites to select molecules.

Dr. Pert explains that the receptors floating on the cell's oily outer surface have roots that go deep into the cellular cytoplasm. Technically, the roots are known as second messengers. Once the receptor is activated, molecules inside the cell respond with a dance of their own. A lively event follows in which molecules signal one another, and enzymatic reactions zip right along. With 3,870 different enzymes catalogued in the human genome, it becomes clear that some sort of organization must control which enzymes are active at a particular time. This brings us to a discussion of the molecules that excite receptors.

Receptors and Their Ligands

Receptors are specific for one particular chemical, and they contain tiny keyholes that exactly fit the shape of the molecule they are seeking. They hover in position with an "arm" extending into the fluid between cells waiting for the appropriate chemical to swim past. Receptors function as sensing devices that scan for the specific chemical needed to energize the cell. Once encountered, the receptor locks onto the target molecule. The chemicals that receptors lock onto are known as ligands, and they can be vitamins, minerals, amino acids, peptides, hormones, or proteins. Each receptor is attracted to a specific ligand—one with the correct electromagnetic vibration and shape that fits snugly into the receptor's active site.

The term *neurotransmitters* originally described small molecules that activate brain cells (neurons), but they have other important functions. Communication between neurons is a one-way street with traffic flowing from a transmitting neuron to a receiving one. Neurotransmitters are released from the transmitting neuron, enter a tiny gap between neurons known as the synapse, and are then bound by receptors on the receiving neuron. This is a highly selective process, with receptors being flooded with thousands of chemical signals at a given time. In order to keep traffic flowing and not clog the synapse with surplus neurotransmitters, the transmitting neuron can recall surplus neurotransmitters. This is called *reuptake* and is a mechanism targeted by many neuroleptic drugs including some used to control stress and depression. For example, a newer class of antidepressants are called serotonin reuptake inhibitors or SSRIs. These drugs raise the concentration of the neurotransmitter serotonin in the synapse by blocking its reuptake by the transmitting neuron.

Neurotransmitters are active outside the brain, stimulating peripheral nerves, including those in most organs. They are also very active in the immune system. Having a "gut feeling" about something is actually the neurotransmitters in your intestines doing the talking. Moreover, neurotransmitters aren't the only chemicals that activate brain cells. A typical neuron has millions of receptors on its surface that scan for steroid hormones and peptides (small strings of amino acids).

Peptides

Ninety-five percent of ligands, including many hormones that interact with receptors, are peptides. Some of the most important are enkephalins and endorphins, which are your natural pain killers. Others are substance P, oxytocin, insulin, gut peptides, corticotropin-releasing factor (CRF), and bradykinin. Peptides are involved in regulating nearly all of life's processes. Peptide release in the brain is affected by behavior, and brain peptides in turn regulate immune function. Most importantly, the exchange of information is bidirectional, so what you are thinking and feeling has a real impact on your wellness and vice versa.

Norman Cousins shocked the medical community when he recovered from a life-threatening illness in 1964 by using the power of laughter. His remarkable recovery was recounted in *Anatomy of an Illness*. Cousins, a well-known journalist, had discovered the power of mind/body interaction. His story inspired scientists including Dr. Pert to research neuropeptides and their interaction with the immune system. She and other scientists found that there is widespread neuropeptide receptor distribution in the emotional processing centers of the brain structures and also throughout organ systems of the body. Dr. Pert dubbed these peptides the "molecules of emotion," and they are located in every cell in your body. You can lock into this power every day of your life. Connecting with these molecules is the first thing you must do during meditation.

Hormones

We'll talk about several hormones including the sex hormones in chapters 6 and 7, but in this chapter we are interested in the effect of stress on the hormone cortisol. Hormone release is a carefully controlled step-by-step process.

Stress activates a part of the brain known as the hypothalamic-pituitary-adrenal (HPA) axis, and it releases peptides including corticotropin-releasing factor or CRF. These peptides serve as the central coordinators for neuroendocrine (hormone), immune, and behavioral responses to stress. CRF is specifically concerned with the adrenal glands, and it stimulates the adrenal-activating peptide adrenocorticotropic hormone or ACTH to release the hormones cortisol and glucagon. These hormones frame the stress response by altering behavior, triggering release of multiple peptides, and changing involuntary nervous system functions such as digestion. Cortisol and glucagon also change the way glucose and oxygen are utilized by the brain and muscles to get you out of danger.

In addition to cortisol and glucagon, the adrenal glands secrete the neurotransmitters epinephrine (adrenaline) and norepinephrine (noradrenaline). The two neurotransmitters stimulate the brain and activate the fight-or-flight response with which we are all too familiar. The effect of all this molecular exchange is a series of lifesaving events that protect you from infection or injury. However, chronic stress puts the body on high alert, sacrificing other events that are needed to promote health and longevity.

Glucagon bumps up the conversion of muscle tissue to glucose to provide a ready source of fuel for molecules engaged in the stress battle. A glucose surplus eventually leads to weight gain and inappropriate insulin response. During nonstress periods, glucagon is balanced by insulin, which keeps blood sugar under control and promotes uptake of proteins into muscles. However, during stressful periods, the glucagon/insulin balance is tipped and protein breakdown (catabolism) is increased. High levels of cortisol enhance this effect. By far the worst effect of high cortisol is aging.

Cortisol and Aging

Cortisol affects every cell of your body and your central nervous system, activating protective defense mechanisms to save your life. However, persistent elevation of cortisol disrupts homeostasis by interfering with hormone, immune, brain, and nerve function. For example, high-stress states produce lapses in short-term memory, affect appetite, and weaken your immune response. You know how easy it is to get a cold or other ailment when you've been highly stressed.

In an amazing feedback loop, rising levels of certain neurotransmitters, hormones, and peptides alert the brain that the stress is still there, and the adrenals kick in more cortisol. This is extremely useful when we are threatened with bodily harm or attack by microbes, but it's of little use when we're stuck in traffic on the freeway. Eventually high circulating cortisol levels deplete the adrenal glands of cortisol reserves and initiate an unremitting stress cycle that ultimately leads to adrenal exhaustion and chronic disease development.

Effects of Stress on Your Brain and Body

Cortisol has been dubbed the age-accelerating hormone. The main function of cortisol is to reduce inflammation in case of injury, and, indeed, the drug cortisone is used for that purpose. However, as we age, cortisol levels rise. The more stressful our lifestyle and the poorer our diet, the higher the cortisol levels. High cortisol levels are directly related to 11 major factors in aging:

1. Collagen and elastin protein breakdown in skin, joint, bone, and muscle tissue
2. Memory loss and nervous system damage
3. Decreased immune function
4. Increased pro-inflammatory signaling factors called *eicosanoids*
5. Fat metabolism disorders reflected in elevated triglyceride, total cholesterol, and low good-to-bad cholesterol ratio
6. Body fluid retention and high blood pressure
7. Decreased hormone signaling capability
8. Increased hypoglycemia and sugar cravings due to increased insulin levels
9. Increased inflammation due to allergies, asthma, and arthritis
10. Skin problems, wrinkles, acne, psoriasis, seborrhea, and alopecia (hair loss)
11. Decreased cognitive function

High Cortisol and Hormone Imbalances

Increased cortisol alters the function of other hormones including growth hormone, insulin, thyroid-stimulating hormone, and sex hormones. Neurotransmitters and neuropeptides are also affected. The immune system receives these chemical signals and communicates messages back to the central nervous system, with some cytokines directly affecting the brain. The intimate communication alters immune response, inflammation, and pain perception. That's why constant stress produces illness, most notably head and body aches. Stress and elevated cortisol levels also cause skin disorders such as acne, seborrhea, hair loss, skin aging, and wrinkles. Moreover, stress contributes to reproductive problems including premenstrual syndrome (PMS), menopausal symptoms, low libido, and lack of fertility.

Appendix A tells you how to get a saliva test kit for determining your cortisol and other hormone levels. *The Anti-Aging Solution* gives you the guidance you need to reduce stress and balance your hormones.

Stress and Free Radicals

Constant stress produces burgeoning numbers of free radicals as your mitochondria amp up production of energy to support the molecules involved in the stress response. Your body, especially if it's not well nourished, cannot neutralize the massive numbers of radicals produced during high-stress periods.

Cytokines are important mediators of inflammation. They are also involved in protein catabolism (breakdown). Like the stress hormones, certain cytokines including TNFα are associated with loss of muscle protein and increased synthesis of inflammatory proteins such as C-reactive protein. Stress ages you by damaging your genes, proteins, carbohydrates, and lipids.

Action Steps: How to Control Stress

Each day in the life of your genes begins with stress-control methods. You can choose what works best for you and fits within your personal belief system. Now that you understand that your cells communicate in a harmonious melody, you can help orchestrate the music by sending them messages from your emotions.

Be Aware of a New Day

Spend a few extra minutes after wakening just to become aware of your body. This means checking to see how you feel and being grateful for what your cells were doing during the night. As you slept, they were storing up energy and busily humming away. Hormone levels follow 12-hour patterns and so do levels of peptides and enzymes. Be grateful for the warmth and comfort of your bed and your health. Welcome the new day and think about the positive things that will happen.

If you have chronic pain when you wake in the morning, you can use this time to send messages to the pain centers of your brain to increase your natural opiate-like painkilling endorphins. Work to create a positive image of the health you are building and how you will overcome disability. Take several deep breaths, stretch your limbs, then roll out of bed.

Breathe Deeply and Slowly

Ancient and modern healing arts share a common practice of correct breathing. Meditation, yoga, qi gong, tai chi, and Pilates teach you the importance of drawing air into your core (Pilates) or lower dantian (qi gong), or third chakra (yoga). This is the area behind your navel, considered the center of energy or fire.

Accessing it requires tightening the lower abdominal (transverse abdominal) or "seat belt" muscles and drawing air downward toward your lower spine. As you do this, you will be using the back of your rib cage to fill your lungs with air. Most people deeply inhale by pushing the rib cage out toward the front of their body. This increases tension on the shoulders. With lower abdominal breathing, the shoulders naturally drop and the collarbone widens.

Inhale deeply and slowly through your nose and exhale by slowly blowing air out through your slightly open mouth. Purse your lips slightly as if you were blowing the puffy white seeds from a dandelion. Breathe deeply three or four times. Do this deep breathing exercise frequently throughout the day.

Meditate Every Day

Once out of bed, find a comfortable place of solitude to meditate. Meditation has been practiced and perfected as a process for healing and restoring mind/body. All ancient healing methods used meditation as a time to connect with one's inner being and activate the powerful healing ability of the body.

Meditation was developed by traditional healers within the context of prayer, whereas in holistic medicine it is employed as a healing technique independent of one's spiritual and cultural beliefs. Most of us, however, find that meditation leads to a natural connection with the universe as we gather energy from the environment around us.

Modern science has now validated the practice of meditation as the way to connect with the molecules of our emotions. Scientists have found that meditation changes the frequency of brain waves and allows us to access other levels of awareness. For example, when Buddhist monks are meditating and cloistered priests or nuns are at prayer, electrical waves in their brain's awareness center (posterior superior parietal lobe) show strikingly low activity. This part of the brain, dubbed the orientation association area, provides a sharp distinction between our body and our surroundings. Slowing this center down promotes a feeling of peace and oneness with the universe that can be powerful medicine in today's hectic world.

According to Hemlata Pokharna, Ph.D., Department of Medicine, University of Chicago, "The main purpose of meditation is to bring steadiness to the mind, which usually remains disturbed as it is constantly stimulated by the sense organs, sense objects, and countless desires." Meditation gradually releases the mind from disturbance or confusion and moves it toward greater calmness, clarity, and focus. Dr. Pokharna lists these functions of meditation:

Curb existing thoughts and block new thoughts from entering the mind, so that one becomes "thoughtless."

Retain only desired thoughts in the mind—those that enhance healing.

Simply observe thoughts as they pass through your mind as if you are an impartial witness, while blocking emotional "knee jerk" responses. As you practice this you'll find that certain images bring instant calmness while others demand a response. It's the latter that you need to suppress. Busy brains have a hard time with this one but it's well worth the effort.

Thoughtlessness allows you to communicate fully with your cells and to create a vision of health and longevity. You use your mind to access the healing wisdom of your cells and energize them. Thus, you can tap into the natural force within to overcome ill health or disability and promote longevity. Meditation will take you out of any emotional hurts or insults you have suffered and alleviate a desire for anger and revenge. It also gives you the ability to release excessive information from your mind.

Meditation has several components, the first of which is breathing. Using the technique given above, take in several deep breaths to pull energy into your lower abdominal area. As you exhale, slowly release any concerns or thoughts. It will take daily work, but soon you will be able to free your mind with little effort. We suggest you get books or tapes on meditation that can guide you. Practice meditation at least twice a day: upon awakening and before going to sleep. During the day, go to a secluded spot to meditate if possible. At the very least, take frequent breathing breaks throughout the day.

Now, you have begun your day with time to experience a place of perfect peace and understanding. You may have had to get up a half hour earlier, but you need this time to get your mind and body synchronized. It is essential that you ground yourself before heading out for the day.

Stretch Every Day

After meditating, spend 10 minutes stretching. There are many books on how to stretch including those on workouts, yoga, tai chi, and qi gong. Some are listed in the resources section in the back of this book. If you exercise in the morning, do your stretching just before you exercise. Chapter 5 features anti-aging exercises, and you'll find the breathing techniques you learned in this chapter will be used in exercise as well.

Prepare for Your Day

The rest of your morning routine should coincide with the excellent start you have made. Let your mind, hormones, and immune system establish connections that will buffer you against the day's stressful events. Take this time to feel good about yourself, not to plan your day. As you move into the next few activities, you'll find your creative mind goes to work. Many people find that solutions to problems or creative ideas suddenly emerge while they are in the shower. Exercise control over these ideas. Let them mature as you eat breakfast and head out the door. Use commuting time to listen to music or inspirational tapes, or read on the train. Avoid using your cell phone, especially when driving. As you move through the other events in your day, always work to keep stress under control.

Relax

Relaxation is another anti-aging technique that accesses the healing ability of your cells. Emmett Miller, M.D., a well-known expert on deep relaxation/guided imagery, is a pioneer in the practice of mind/body medicine. According to Dr. Miller, "Deep relaxation can be dramatically effective in relieving symptoms such as inflammation, anxiety, and muscle tension. It can be a lifesaver when dealing with stress and life crises. By relieving tension, deep relaxation improves circulation and speeds up healing." Dr. Miller has produced excellent books and relaxation tapes that you will find helpful. These are listed in the resources section of this book.

Taking frequent breaks throughout the day for stress relief through breathing, stretching, relaxation, and meditation will extend your healthy years and add to your quality of life.

CHAPTER 4

Step 2: Nourish Your Genes

A man may esteem himself happy when that which is his food is also his medicine.

—Henry David Thoreau

A Festival of Food

Food has been at the center of social events in times of joy and sorrow for millennia. It has served as the focal point for gatherings of family and friends, and special days of seasonal festivals have been set aside just to celebrate with special foods. Harvest festivals highlighting the season's bounty have featured corn, beans, berries, fish, and poultry, among other foods. Religious holidays throughout the world are celebrated with traditional meals. Food has even been used to deliver a message such as espousing love and friendship with chocolate on Valentine's Day or delivering cookies to welcome a new neighbor. It is firmly ingrained that food satisfies our deepest psychological and social needs, but what about our physical need for nourishment?

The drive to find food is second only to that of staying alive. Throughout most of human history, a major proportion of time has been spent obtaining and preparing food. Whole families engaged in this pursuit until well into the twentieth century when grocery stores began providing most of our food. Still, homemade and made from scratch lend a unique importance to food gifts, and the satisfaction of growing things to eat has persisted, as evidenced by the popularity of small home gardens. Yet there has been an alarming distortion between satisfying our physical, psychological, and social needs for food and its preparation and consumption. And it's killing us.

The Disappearing Family Meal

Traditionally, at dinnertime family members gathered to discuss daily events and enjoy a good meal. However, the daily ceremony of family dining has disappeared in many homes as increasing outside activities necessitate flexible mealtimes. It has been replaced by a grab-and-feed mentality with mindless shopping for food that most quickly and easily satisfies hunger. Parents stop at a drive-up window and grab a bucket of fatty food that will quiet little ones in the car while satiating older children heading for sports practice. Such food provides short-term sustenance but does little to nourish the cells that sustain us.

Portion Size—A Call to Action

The popularity of fast foods and the convenience of ready-to-eat-meals have largely replaced traditional meal planning and preparation. Such quick-fix meals on wheels are less nutritious and contain too many calories. Leading nutritionists have often maintained that diminished senses of taste and smell lead people to eat more. Fatty foods that are bland and tasteless will drive us to eat larger servings in search of more flavor sensation. Consequently, portion size has increased dramatically, as consumers have mistakenly associated food value with quantity rather than quality.

Supersize meals have become so popular that even diet foods come in larger portions. Lean Cuisine frozen dinners now come in a "hearty portion" that weighs 50 percent more than the original, and Weight Watchers now advertises larger portions. In the 1950s, McDonald's offered only one size of french fries. It's now the "small" size and weighs just one-third that of the largest size. Recipes have also grown in portion size. A check of recipes in cookbooks that have been mainstays for 40 or 50 years reveals that the same list of ingredients now supplies only half the servings. Do portion sizes really affect how much people eat?

Barbara Rolls, Ph.D., and colleagues from the Department of Nutritional Sciences, Pennsylvania State University, answered this question when they enrolled 51 men and women in a lunch program that offered varying portion sizes of macaroni and cheese. One day during each of 4 weeks the study participants were given 2½-, 3-, 3¾-, or 5-cup portions.

Half of the people were served their portions on a plate. The other half received portions in a serving dish and were told to take as much as they wanted. In all cases, the subjects ate all that was offered regardless of how it was served. The subjects consumed 30 percent more (160 calories) when offered the largest portion compared to the smallest. Body weight, body mass index (BMI), gender, or being on a "diet" didn't make a difference in the amount each person chose to eat.

The researchers demonstrated with this study that appetite was determined solely by how much was on the plate. Apparently the test subjects chose to override their internal satiety signals. Are portion sizes increasing because we're hungrier or because we don't know when we're full because the food we're eating doesn't satisfy us?

Think about your own meal behavior. Do you tend to push away from the table when you're full or when your plate is empty? Do you frequently serve yourself second helpings? If you're over 40 and moderately active, you need about half the calories you consumed as a 20-year-old. Many people over 60 can do nicely with two well-balanced meals a day, and some 80-year-olds stay healthy and youthful with one well-balanced meal a day. Lighter snacks of vegetables, nuts, or high-quality proteins sustain energy between meals. As quantity of food decreases, it becomes exceedingly important that it has the best nutritional quality. Unfortunately, we're getting fatter as portion sizes increase. Obesity is aging us at an unprecedented rate.

Moreover, intake of snack foods and beverages has increased dramatically in modern countries while that of high-fiber and micronutrient-dense foods such as vegetables, fruit, and whole grains has decreased.

Eating Our Way to Premature Aging

A wave of recent lawsuits blaming fast-food outlets for causing obesity plus the enormous popularity of such books as *Fast Food Nation* have put fast and snack foods under intense scrutiny. As the typical Western diet with its fast-food phenomena has spread to other countries, there has been a parallel increase in obesity. There is a well-documented link between being overweight and aging.

In a new study published in the *Annals of Internal Medicine,* Anna Peeters, Ph.D., and colleagues analyzed data from 3,457 men and women enrolled in the Framingham Heart Study. They found that overweight 40-year-olds who had never smoked were likely to die 3 years sooner than their slimmer counterparts—a decrease in life span that's equivalent to that seen in normal-weight smokers. The combination of smoking and being overweight shortened life span by an incredible 13 years.

Animal research suggests that aging is associated with progressive declines in normal metabolism and response to dietary factors. And as nations become more industrialized, adopting a more sedentary lifestyle and eating easy-to-obtain but less nutritious food, incidence of overweight will only increase.

A staggering 90 percent of aging conditions stem from being overweight. You determined your BMI in chapter 1 as part of assessing your Aging Equation. Now you will see that a normal BMI is strongly associated with health and longevity. The following figure illustrates the rapid rise in diseases with increasing BMI:

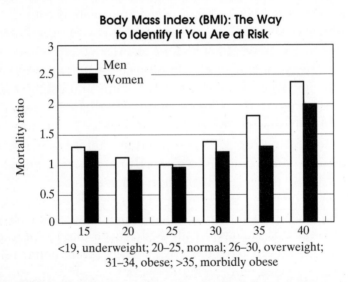

Body Mass Index (BMI): The Way to Identify If You Are at Risk

<19, underweight; 20–25, normal; 26–30, overweight; 31–34, obese; >35, morbidly obese

A BMI between 20 and 25 is considered ideal and is associated with a very low risk of disease. A BMI lower than 19 increases the risk of certain diseases. Note the differences between men and women with the same BMI and risk of disease. Although risk of disease is intensified as BMI increases, men have an even greater chance for developing a life-threatening condition. Obesity and high BMI are implicated in most aging conditions. The goal of the anti-aging menu makeover is to achieve a BMI below 30, which translates into a more youthful body composition and a reduced risk of disease. Mary's case illustrates that

Health Consequences Associated with a BMI Greater Than 27	
⇨ Insulin resistance	⇨ Cardiovascular problems
⇨ Non-insulin-dependent diabetes mellitus	⇨ Gallstones
	⇨ Cholecystitis
⇨ Hypertension	⇨ Respiratory dysfunction
⇨ Dyslipidemia	⇨ Certain forms of cancer

although the goal of anti-aging eating isn't specifically weight loss, good nutrition does in fact lead to a lowered BMI and weight loss:

I came to the Giampapa Institute in February 2002 because I needed help in losing weight before having knee surgery. Dr. Giampapa first discussed the impact of weight on aging and aging conditions including knee problems, which had made my surgery necessary. He did a complete anti-aging work-up that included health questionnaire, blood work, diet analysis, and hormone balance. He then provided me with a complete program that included an eating plan geared more to anti-aging than weight loss. It included eating five small meals a day totaling 1,200 calories. He also put me on supplements, prescribed an exercise program, and added a hormone-balancing plan.

In 2 years, I've lost a total of 50 pounds. I've been exercising as well as watching what I eat. My BMI was 32 and now it's 23, which is ideal. I have been walking, taking spin classes at a local gym, and swimming three or four times per week. Now that I am more active, I can maintain my weight on 1,500 calories per day. I see remarkable changes in my body shape due to the eating plan and exercise. I have improved energy levels, better retention/memory skills, and feel better overall.

Healthy Eating

Brightly colored foods and whole grains that contain a variety of vitamins, minerals, and phytochemicals satisfy your appetite, whereas those that are nutrient deficient and monochromatic don't (e.g., processed foods). This is the core concept of our anti-aging diet plan. Changing how you feed your genes is the best way to improve your health and longevity, and it's the easiest thing to do.

You will have to give more time and thought to meal planning, shopping, storing, and preparing your meals. And this may mean that you have to reprioritize the important events in your life. If you have children, they will be learning a valuable lesson on how to live a longer, healthier life. Besides, you'll actually save food dollars. It's a common misconception that buying healthier foods is costlier.

Do Healthier Foods Cost More?

Doctors at a family-based obesity treatment program in New York conducted a yearlong study of 31 families with obese 8- to 12-year-olds. A 20-week dietary and behavior instruction period at the beginning of the study emphasized eating nutrient-dense foods instead of fast and processed foods. Choosing nutrient-dense foods was reinforced during counseling sessions and by keeping careful records of foods eaten, daily food cost, calorie intake, and percentage of calories from proteins, carbohydrates, and fats. The researchers collected these data at the beginning of the trial, at 6 months, and at 12 months.

The weight loss among parents and children was impressive. Children's weight was reduced significantly (6.7 percent at 6 months, 10.3 percent at 12 months) while their parents lost 6.7 percent of their weight at 6 months and 5.3 percent after 1 year. Average daily caloric intake for both parents and children dropped from 1,881 at baseline to 1,412 at 6 months and 1,338 at 1 year.

Most importantly, servings from unhealthy food decreased over the year, dropping from 34.7 percent of foods eaten at the beginning of the study to 18.6 percent at the end. As for cost, 6 months into the study the food budget stayed pretty much the same. However, it dropped dramatically by the end of the year. The cost per ounce of healthy foods was greater, but the cost per calorie consumed between healthy and unhealthy foods was the same. Since the number of daily calories consumed was less, overall cost for foods dropped. It takes more calories from unhealthy foods to satisfy your appetite while micronutrient-dense foods containing vitamins, minerals, fiber, and essential fatty acids provide greater satiety.

This study demonstrates that switching from fast and snack foods to choices that are more healthful can actually save on the family food budget while fighting the obesity problem. Well-designed longer-term studies would no doubt show both health benefits and cost savings when people follow a healthy diet for many years. Nevertheless, we can rely on the long-term studies that document disease resistance and alleviation of disease conditions when people eat a healthy diet.

How Good Is Your Diet?

Data from the longest-running studies of thousands of people, many of them health professionals, have shown that those eating the most fruits and vegetables have lower rates of cancer, diabetes, and heart disease. Yet the latest food surveys indicate that 80 percent of us do not eat the minimum 5 servings of fruits and vegetables a day. The latest evidence suggests that most men need to bump up their consumption of fruits and vegetables to 7 or 9 daily servings, which we suggest in our meal plans. We'll show you how easy it is to get these servings later in this chapter. Fruits and vegetables supply most of our anti-aging nutrients; they're rich in flavor and their satiety factor is high. Leading experts have repeatedly pointed to poor diet as the cause of chronic conditions that are prematurely aging us. The biggest culprit is sugar.

The Sugar Trap

Sugars perform many vital functions in the body in addition to providing the major source of energy as glucose. Complex sugars adorn the exposed surface of membrane receptors, flagging down passing chemicals as described in chapter 3. Other sugars such as glucosamine protect joints. These functional sugars can be damaged by oxidative stress, leading to crippling conditions such as osteoarthritis. However, we're going to focus on glucose and what happens when it's oxidized by free radicals.

Oxidized glucose coats the surface of proteins such as collagen, hemoglobin, and albumin, preventing them from functioning. Scientists call this process *glycation*. Collagen is the most plentiful protein in your body and the one most affected by glycation. Skin, blood, and lymph vessels, joints, tendons, ligaments, and internal organs are comprised of collagen. Most aging conditions are linked to glycation including

- Memory loss: sugar coating of brain neurons (brain cells)
- Clinical depression: disruption of neurotransmitter function
- Reduced stress adaptation: damaged cortisol receptors
- Hormone imbalances: increased unbound or free cortisol
- Skin wrinkling and sagging: collagen glycation
- Impaired immune function: damage to thymus gland, lymphatic tissue, and immune cells

- Allergies, leaky gut syndrome, and irritable bowel disorders: impaired gastrointestinal function and decreased digestive capacity

Persistent sleepiness after meals, which is common among older people, is one of the first signs that sugar problems exist. Although it's not surprising for this symptom to occur among those who have passed their sixth or seventh decade, it should not happen to those in their twenties, provided they are getting enough sleep. Eating a meal high in carbohydrates, especially white flour products, is the cause of the problem.

The typical Western diet, which is loaded with white flour products, refined sugars, snack and fast foods, quickly turns into glucose. The ultimate result of a high-glucose load—a very stressful event for your body—is glycation. The worst part is that every doughnut, candy bar, and soda adds a toxic dose of glucose that winds up sticking to your proteins. The first place this shows up is on your face: from teenage blemishes to middle-age wrinkles. You'll learn more about this in chapter 7. Glycation is a progressive process, and eventually destructive by-products called *advanced glycation end products* (AGEs) are formed. AGEs cause many aging conditions.

Protein and Enzyme Damage

DNA encodes new proteins for the various functions they perform. The codes for manufacturing proteins occupy nearly one-fourth of your genetic material. Some are enzymes that control metabolism, others are structural components of the body, and still others are the small peptides that chaperone larger functional proteins and help attract their appropriate cofactors.

When DNA is damaged, it produces structural abnormalities in proteins that alter their function. Furthermore, glycation causes cross-links to form that make normally pliable proteins stiff and unyielding. Antioxidant-rich foods and antioxidant supplements protect DNA and proteins as well as other key molecules such as membrane fatty acids.

Effects of Insulin

We showed how refined carbohydrate intake raises levels of the stress hormone cortisol. Now we're going to explain how sugar intake affects the hormone insulin and how this alters genetic expression, contributing to several age-related conditions.

Insulin, which is secreted by the pancreas, is the chief hormone that controls metabolism. It affects virtually every cell in your body. It stimulates anabolic (building) reactions for carbohydrates, proteins, and fats. However, its effects are most pronounced in fat tissue, muscle, and the liver. The short-term effects of insulin are to reduce blood sugar by increasing its uptake into cells and to conserve the body's fuel supplies. It also helps regulate gene transcription and cellular replication. The effects of insulin are balanced by another pancreatic hormone, glucagon, which stimulates catabolic (breakdown) reactions and can be thought of as antagonistic to insulin.

Effects of Foods on Hormones

Food

↓

Macronutrients
(carbohydrates, proteins, and fat)

Good Ratios	Poor Ratios
Glucagon maximizes fat burning	Insulin minimizes fat burning
Good Eicosanoids	Bad Eicosanoids
OPTIMUM HEALTH	POOR HEALTH

The ratio between carbohydrates, proteins, and fats from the diet determines the ratio of insulin to glucagon. A high ratio of insulin to glucagon increases fat storage and generation of fatty acid metabolites that promote aging and aging conditions.

A staggering 200,000 insulin receptors can be found in the membranes of cells targeted by this hormone. As insulin locks onto these receptors, it affects cellular enzymes that store proteins, carbohydrates, and fats. Liver and fat cells contain the most insulin receptors because they process carbohydrates and fats into stored fuels. Insulin also interacts with other hormones, primarily cortisol and dehydroepiandrosterone (DHEA), an anti-aging adrenal hormone, plus various growth factors such as insulin-like growth factor 1 (IGF-1), which also mediates fat storage.

Insulin Resistance

A disturbing health trend toward decreased sensitivity of receptors for binding insulin has scientists worried about the myriad of diseases that could be triggered. Such receptor insensitivity is known as insulin resistance and is part of a broader syndrome of disorders that include obesity, high blood pressure, and high cholesterol. These four disorders are closely linked and are sometimes referred to as syndrome X. Each occupies one leg of the X, and, depending on severity, can make up a recipe for heart disease. Insulin resistance alone leads to several life-threatening disorders.

Insulin Resistance and Effects on Aging

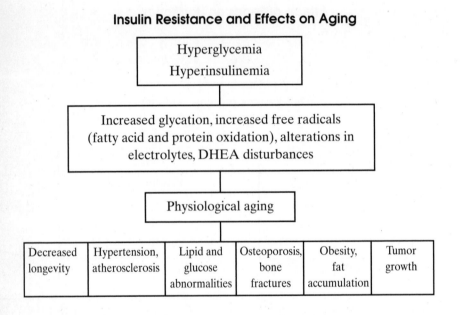

Insulin resistance also increases glycation, and its effect on hormones is as devastating as it is on proteins. The key hormones that keep your body youthful—insulin, glucagon, DHEA, growth hormone, and IGF-1—do not function effectively when they are coated in sugar.

The tendency for insulin resistance is programmed into your genes and may have helped primitive humans survive during periods of starvation by increasing the storage of energy-rich foods. In today's industrialized world, insulin resistance represents a modern scourge because it is greatly aggravated by obesity and physical inactivity. Insulin resistance accompanied by upper body fat, particularly in women, increases the risk of diabetes.

Insulin resistance causes release of too much insulin by the pancreas. Many doctors regard it as the primary factor in diabetes, which is linked with premature aging. Insulin resistance affects the sex hormones as well. In women, increased levels of androgens such as testosterone increase insulin and insulin resistance. Oddly, just the opposite is true for men: they have less insulin resistance when they have high levels of testosterone.

Insulin resistance also occurs in children, with girls being about 35 percent more prone to it than boys. Terry Wilklin, Ph.D., director of the EarlyBird Research Centre in Plymouth, England, studied obesity in more than 300 schoolchildren. Physical activity and weight gain were factored into the insulin resistance equation, so the findings related to gender were objective.

As we grow older, we become less efficient at digestion and absorption of nutrients. Unhealthy foods that we once tolerated have a broader impact as we approach midlife and beyond. At the same time, our internal antioxidant systems become less effective at eliminating free radicals and toxins. A buildup of the enzyme monoamine oxidase in the brain reduces the activity of the important neurotransmitters serotonin, epinephrine, and norepinephrine. These "happy chemicals" not only maintain mental stability but serotonin also reins in appetite. Consequently, its precursors, L-tryptophan and 5-hydroxytryptophan, have been successfully used in weight-loss programs. In an unremitting cycle, overweight people have elevated levels of monoamine oxidase,

Age-Related Changes in Nutrient, Free Radical, and Brain Enzyme Values

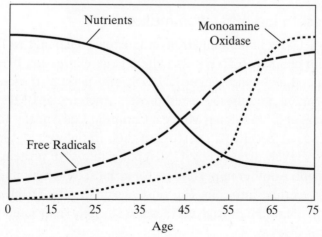

resulting in low serotonin and an increased urge to overeat. Depression often accompanies this cycle.

Insulin Resistance, IGF-1, and Breast Cancer

Recent studies have shown that insulin resistance, hyperinsulinemia, and an increased concentration of IGF-1 are risk factors for breast cancer. The risk is increased with high levels of free estradiol and free testosterone. In obese postmenopausal women, fatty tissues produce an excess of free fatty acids and TNFα, both of which may increase insulin resistance. Fat tissue is also a storage site for estrogen—a major reason that obesity increases the risk of breast cancer.

A Western diet with its emphasis on fatty foods, refined carbohydrates, and saturated fats increases the deleterious effects of high levels of the sex hormones. Consequently, Italian researchers studied the impact of dietary change among postmenopausal women with higher than normal testosterone levels. Dietary intervention among 104 healthy women with high levels of free testosterone (which can ultimately be converted into estrogen) resulted in significant weight loss and increased binding of free testosterone and estrogen to proteins. Waist-to-hip ratio, cholesterol, and fasting blood glucose levels were all reduced. The diet was designed to reduce insulin resistance and cellular uptake of circulating hormones, particularly in postmenopausal women with high levels of androgens. The diet used is similar to the one recommended in our 5-Step Plan: low in animal fat and refined carbohydrates yet rich in low-glycemic foods, healthy monounsaturated and omega-3 polyunsaturated fatty acids, and phytoestrogens.

Insulin Resistance and Inflammation

The role of TNFα in inflammation and increased damage to DNA was explored in chapter 2. TNFα also alters gene expression by changing protein encoding by messenger RNA. Scientists refer to such proteins as TNF proteins, and these altered proteins increase as BMI increases. Researchers at Cedars-Sinai Medical Center in Los Angeles found that when obese subjects lost 26 percent of their initial weight, their TNFα and mRNA levels dropped by 42 percent, while TNF protein dropped by 54 percent. Another important factor is that TNFα inhibits uptake of serum triglycerides into cells. This raises serum levels of triglycerides in obese individuals. High triglycerides are strongly associated with cardiovascular disease.

Aging, Cognitive Function, and Obesity

The Framingham Heart Study, which began in 1948, has yielded a bumper crop of information on nutrition and aging. Boston University's Merrill Elias, M.P.H., Ph.D., and his colleagues analyzed 18 years of data gathered from 551 men and 872 women to see if obesity and hypertension might affect mental performance over time. According to Dr. Elias, "The results indicated that persons who are chronically obese have a higher risk of lowered mental ability—all other things being equal."

The researchers noted that men appear more susceptible to obesity-linked decline in brain power, possibly because they tend to accumulate fat in their midsection. Since obesity is strongly associated with high blood pressure, high cholesterol, and diabetes, perhaps it isn't surprising that the association with decreased mental ability was found. Other studies have shown a greater susceptibility to anxiety and depression with midsection obesity. The association between midsection obesity and estrogen dominance in men that results in cognitive and neurological impairment will be further explored in chapter 7. While central adiposity in women is strongly associated with insulin resistance and diabetes, it does not appear to be as strongly linked to cognitive decline.

Nutrition and Immunity

It has been known for centuries that diet and immunity are linked. Historical accounts have suggested a relationship between famine and epidemics because periods of famine were usually followed by widespread infection. More recently, large epidemiological studies have shown a relationship between malnutrition and heightened risk of bacterial, viral, and protozoal infections. Since the 1970s, numerous studies have confirmed that nutrient deficiencies impair immune response and lead to frequent severe infections. Low intakes of protein and micronutrient deficiencies have the most pronounced effects. Too little protein causes abnormalities in immune response including decreased cell-mediated immunity, cytokine release, decreased antibody response to vaccination, and decreased lymphocyte proliferation.

Being overweight is unquestionably the single most important factor in how quickly you will age and suffer from age-related conditions. And while anti-aging eating doesn't focus on weight loss, you will naturally lose weight as you follow the 5-Step Plan in this book.

Action Steps: Nourish Your Genes

By now you have no doubt recognized the connection between what you eat and your personal Aging Equation as influenced by obesity and high BMI. This is unquestionably the number one issue you face in preventing or retarding the hazards of aging. You may have already discovered that in many cases you must cut through cultural and societal barriers to achieve your dietary goals. Since how you have been eating is intimately linked with your personality and lifestyle, your menu makeover equates with a personality and lifestyle makeover. You will be changing your total concept of remaining healthy.

We encourage you to embrace our message for a healthy life. Avoid overweight and you can avoid most age-associated diseases. The foods we suggest cross cultural boundaries and are in fact the dietary preferences for those who live long, healthy lives. The details of how these foods help you avoid aging are discussed below.

Dietary choices include appropriate portion sizes, the frequency of meals, and the correct order in which to eat foods rich in proteins, carbohydrates, and fats. We also use color to select foods. For example, tan/brown carbohydrates are better for you than those that are white. Protein-rich foods are important to stave off aging. Using the correct oils can spare your cardiovascular system and help you lose weight.

You will learn that food pigments called phytonutrients can be grouped into five food color categories (yellow/orange, green, purple/blue, tan, and white), and each class gives you a special health benefit. Using the meal planner guide and daily meal plans, you will become proficient at choosing colorful foods for visual appeal and health-promoting benefits.

Eating for Anti-Aging Benefits

Anti-aging eating is very different from a weight-loss plan. Whereas the latter focuses on losing pounds, anti-aging eating is a lifestyle modification that alters your body composition so that you obtain a more youthful ratio of fat to lean muscle. Instead of getting on the scale, try getting into something that's too tight to wear comfortably. If you scored high in either the BMI calculation or caliper measurement, your body needs some work. After following the guidelines in this chapter for 60 days, recalculate your BMI and check your caliper measurement. Then try on those clothes that didn't fit. By focusing on BMI and body composition instead of weight, you will

- Burn calories more efficiently by increasing muscle mass
- Decrease age-related conditions as muscle mass increases
- Improve your quality of life as your body functions better
- Normalize hormone levels and improve the balance between them, thus directly affecting the rate of aging
- Bump up antioxidant levels
- Reduce pain and inflammation
- Improve cellular function

Let's begin the plan that will satisfy nutrient requirements in your cells. There are 10 basic rules in anti-aging eating.

Ten Rules for Anti-Aging Eating

Keep these 10 rules in mind when planning your meals. This is a quick checklist, and more detail on each rule follows.

1. Eat selectively.
2. Eat smaller nutritious meals more frequently; don't eat on the run.
3. Choose brown or tan carbohydrates, not white ones.
4. Emphasize protein, concentrating on vegetable sources as much as possible.
5. Eat your protein foods first, followed by nonstarchy vegetables, then carbohydrates.
6. Drink plenty of liquids between meals instead of with them.
7. If you drink alcoholic beverages, do so with meals and in moderation.
8. Choose seasonal fruits and vegetables with the most intense color.
9. Use only high-quality oils.
10. Eat your meals at regular times of the day in a stress-free environment.

Eat selectively. If you are 50 or older or need to lose weight, you should be switching plate size. Instead of a 10-inch dinner plate, use a 7-inch salad plate for dinner. Serve salad on a 5-inch bread-and-butter plate, and use this smallest size for breakfast and lunch.

Serve yourself half the amount of food you ordinarily put onto your plate, and if you are dining out, order appetizers from the menu and split them with a companion. Most restaurants serve main courses that are too much food for anyone over 35 and many who are much younger.

As you have found out, large portions are not a good value, although they may seem so at the time. You will wind up wearing the "added value" around your midsection!

Eat smaller nutritious meals or snacks more frequently. As you get older, your digestive efficiency decreases. Digestion and absorption of food will be improved with this method. Chew your food carefully and focus on flavor. You will be less inclined to overindulge. You will be supplying your cells with energy, protein, and micronutrients that they need to function optimally. You will also be reducing the tendency to snack on less nutrient-dense foods and beverages. Just remember to stop and enjoy these small meals. Don't eat on the run.

Select only tan or brown starches. In choosing carbohydrate-rich starchy foods, make sure they aren't white. Whole-grain breads, cereals, pasta, and rice are anti-aging foods. Their white flour counterparts increase cross-linking of proteins, the process of glycation that we discussed in chapter 2. Other healthy carbohydrate choices are yellow and orange root vegetables such as carrots, winter squash, sweet potatoes, and yams. White potatoes turn into glucose more quickly than sweet potatoes or yams. Peas and corn are starchy nonroot vegetables. Fruit is also a high-carbohydrate food, and there are lots of colors to choose from.

Eat more protein. Fish, poultry, eggs, soft cheese, and lean meat are all good sources of protein. Emphasize vegetable sources from legumes and green vegetables as much as possible. As you grow older, ratios between your intake of protein, carbohydrates, and fat should slowly shift. Proteins supply the necessary raw materials for good genetic repair and maintenance of lean muscle. Overall intake of carbohydrates should be reduced, with the emphasis on complex carbohydrates. It is also important to get your fat servings from healthy oils such as canola, olive, macadamia, flaxseed, and walnut oils. Dramatically reduce your intake of processed and fast foods, working to completely eliminate them.

Eat food in the proper order. Eat protein foods first because they take longer to digest and slow the absorption of sugars from carbohydrate-rich foods. Next, eat your vegetables, and save complex carbohydrates for last. It's best to eat fruit between meals, but if you are eating a fruit and green salad combination, eat it last. Skip desserts after meals or before bedtime. If you want to occasionally enjoy a pastry or other very sweet treat, do so at least 2 hours before eating a meal.

Don't drink liquids with your meals. Water and other liquids dilute digestive enzymes. Ice water is particularly bad as it chills the stomach, reducing its efficiency. A notable exception to this rule is wine. If you drink it, do so with meals.

Drink plenty of liquids between meals. Water should be your beverage of choice, but coffee, tea, and juices all count toward your total fluid intake. A good rule of thumb is to drink in number of ounces half of your body weight in pounds each day. For example, if you weigh 150 pounds, you should drink 75 ounces of fluids each day. Avoid sodas because they contain acids that leach calcium from the system and demineralize tooth enamel. Sodas are a particularly bad idea if you're sick. They contain several teaspoons of sugar, reducing the scavenging ability of white blood cells, plus they increase protein glycation.

Choose fruits and vegetables with the most intense color. The pigments that color fruits and vegetables come from antioxidants and other phytonutrients that boost your defenses against genetic damage and enhance genetic expression.

Use only high-quality oils. Fat-free foods are being less recommended by nutritionists because the fat has often been replaced by various kinds of sugars. You need healthy oils to anchor your cellular receptors and maintain youthful skin. You need to eliminate margarine, hydrogenated oils, fried foods, and processed foods, because they contain trans fats that are being increasingly implicated in chronic disease. Olive, macadamia nut, walnut, sesame, and canola oils are excellent choices, and they take high heat for cooking without adverse effects. Canola, walnut, and macadamia nut oils are rich in helpful omega-3 fatty acids. Flaxseed oil is the richest source of omega-3 fatty acids and can be used in dressings, but you should not cook with it because it breaks down in high heat.

Eat your meals in a stress-free environment. The less distraction you have, the more opportunity you will have to enjoy what you are eating. Eat slowly and you'll be satisfied with less food. You will also improve your digestion and assimilation of food. Eating on the run is the worst thing you can do. Drive-through meals promote a grab-and-feed mentality that does not satisfy your nutritional needs.

Color-Coded Eating

Our menu makeover features foods rich in phytonutrients that have disease-fighting power. Phytonutrients are the buzz among food scientists because these amazing plant chemicals have cancer preventive and gene restorative properties. Moreover, they modify genetic expression and improve cellular metabolism, thus slowing aging and alleviating aging conditions. A diet rich in fruits and vegetables improves bone health and bone metabolism, a concern for aging men as well as women.

Phytonutrients are pigments that give plants their bright colors. Those having similar colors have related disease-fighting properties. Take carrots, for example. The orange color is due to a family known as carotenoids. Other orange vegetables—winter squash or orange fruit such as mango—also contain carotenoids and have similar health-promoting benefits. You avail yourself of these healing chemicals when you choose foods by their color.

Your menu makeover emphasizes foods from the following five color groups:

1. Yellow, orange, bright red—carotenoids
2. Green—sulfur compounds, isothiocyanates, indols
3. Purple, blue, black, magenta—phenolics, flavonoids
4. Tan—phytosterols, phytoestrogens, fiber, saponins
5. White—protein, omega-3 fatty acids, omega-6 fatty acids

The color categories of foods are grouped by how they protect your genes and promote your health and longevity. Each category provides specific antioxidants that are a formidable force against free radicals. In chapter 2 we showed that your body uses a family of antioxidants to protect you. Each food group contains important antioxidants that detoxify free radicals to protect your genes and affect genetic expression in a unique way. The food groups are categorized by color and the antioxidants they contain.

Free radicals and toxins not neutralized by internal antioxidant systems must be eliminated by a cycle of dietary antioxidants. Body fluids are protected by vitamin C and bioflavonoids found in purple/red foods. Membranes are protected by vitamin E (tan foods) and carotenoids (yellow/orange foods). Glutathione is produced from cysteine, vitamins, and minerals (green foods).

Dietary Antioxidants Work Together to Counteract Oxidative Stress

Without the entire complement of antioxidants, some free radicals are not neutralized, leading to an accumulation in the body.

> **Incomplete Detoxification**
> Free radicals from
> radiation, drugs, chemicals,
> and toxic metabolites

Detoxification is Completed by

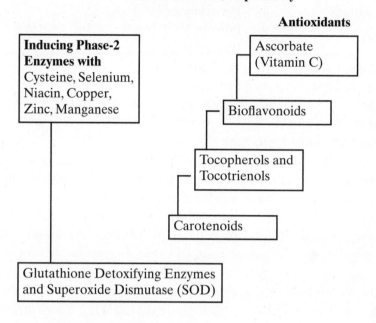

Antioxidants

Inducing Phase-2 Enzymes with Cysteine, Selenium, Niacin, Copper, Zinc, Manganese

Ascorbate (Vitamin C)

Bioflavonoids

Tocopherols and Tocotrienols

Carotenoids

Glutathione Detoxifying Enzymes and Superoxide Dismutase (SOD)

Foods to Protect Genes

- *Colors:* yellow, orange, bright red, yellow/green
- *Phytonutrients:* carotenes: alpha-carotene, beta-carotene, lycopene, lutein, zeaxanthin, vitamin C (in some)
- *Serving size:* ½ cup cooked vegetables or cut-up fruit
- *Servings per day:* 2–3

Vegetables	**Fruit**	**Spices**
Carrots	Apricots	Allspice
Corn	Avocados	Cardamom
Grape leaves	Bananas	Cayenne
Green beans	Cantaloupes	Cinnamom
Hot peppers, cayenne	Grapefruits	Cloves
Lettuce	Kiwi	Curry
Peas	Lemons	Ginger
Pumpkin	Mangos	Nutmeg
Spinach	Nectarines	Saffron
Summer squash	Oranges	Turmeric
Sweet peppers	Papaya	
Tomatoes	Passion fruit	
Turnips	Pears	

Vegetables *(continued)*	**Fruit** *(continued)*
Summer squash	Persimmons
Winter squash	Pineapples
Yams	Pomegranates
Yellow, orange, red	Pomelos
bell peppers, hot	Strawberries
peppers	Tangerines

Why These Foods Are Important

Foods in the yellow/orange/red category are exceptional antioxidants, forming the first line of defense against free radicals generated from physiological stress, air pollution, tobacco smoke, chemical and ultraviolet exposure. Carotenoids—over 600 have been identified—are all fat soluble and have an affinity for cellular membranes. As membrane antioxidants they protect the cell and its organelles, retain membrane fluidity, and improve intercellular communication. They are transported throughout the body, riding piggyback on very low-density (VLDL), low-density (LDL), and high-density (HDL) lipoproteins. Thus, they are uniquely situated to prevent oxidation of lipoproteins, a major factor in atherogenesis.

Carotenes have also been found to reduce angina. Three carotenes—alpha, beta, and gamma—can be converted into vitamin A. Carotenes are photoprotective, anti-inflammatory, cell growth and immune modulators, anti-carcinogenic, and protective of the brain and nervous system. Carotenoid-rich fruits and vegetables are abundant yearlong. Winter vegetables such as squash, yams, sweet potatoes, and pumpkin are high in carotenoid antioxidants and give you extra protection during cold and flu season. Winter antioxidant fruits and vegetables exposed to frost are sweeter and contain higher levels of phytonutrients. That's because sugar works as an antifreeze and phytonutrients protect against environmental stress.

Spices high in carotenoids have the characteristic golden color, are very flavorful, and help you digest your food and speed up a sluggish metabolism. Instead of salt, use pepper and spices liberally, especially when eating protein and foods high in oil content. Ancient cultures have used spices to preserve foods because they retard bacterial, mold, and mildew growth. In Asia, for example, liberal use of curries, garlic, and onions helped preserve food before the days of refrigeration. You need at least three different carotenoid foods every day to preserve your youthfulness.

Foods to Repair Genes, Improve Cellular Nutrients, and Detoxify

- *Colors:* green, green/white
- *Phytonutrients:* sulfur compounds: cysteine, sulphoraphane, isothiocyanates, indoles, and the mineral selenium
- *Serving size:* ½ cup cooked, 1 cup raw
- *Servings per day:* 2–4

Cruciferous Vegetables	Mustard Vegetables	Onion Family	Garlic Family
Asparagus	Arugula	All onions	Fresh garlic
Broccoli	Daikon	Chives	Dried garlic
Broccoli sprouts	Horseradish	Leeks	
Broccoflower	Jicama	Scallions	
Bok choy	Mustard greens	Shallots	
Brussels sprouts	Mustard seed		
Cabbage	Radishes		
Cauliflower	Spices in moderation		
Collards	Sprouts		
Kale			
Kohlrabi			
Rutabaga			
Sauerkraut			
Tatsoi			
Turnips			
Watercress			

Why These Foods Are Important

Foods in this group have a pungent flavor due to their sulfur content. Many grow in the ground or in damp climates. Sulfur is one of the most effective mold deterrents. It is an essential component of DNA repair enzymes. Paul Talaly, M.D., and his team at Johns Hopkins University have shown that the sulfur compounds in this food group, especially broccoli sprouts, are powerful inducers of protective enzymes known as phase 2 detoxifying enzymes including superoxide dismutase and glutathione peroxidase.

Similarly, Edward Giovannucci, Ph.D., a noted epidemiologist from Harvard, and other researchers have found that indoles in cabbage and other crucifers inhibit colorectal, bladder, lung, mouth, throat, stomach, and breast cancers. There is an important distinction between foods in this group and the yellow group, the latter protecting the body by direct free-radical scavenging. So, you need to eat from both groups daily.

Paul Thornalley, Ph.D., University of Essex, United Kingdom, and his team have discovered an important anti-aging property of isothiocyanates. They inhibit enzymes that promote glycation and formation of AGEs. From this work it becomes apparent that green foods are one of your most important allies in the fight against wrinkling and cross-linking of other proteins.

Scottish researchers have reported that indoles and isothiocyanates from cruciferous vegetables protect DNA from damage and stimulate apoptosis in colon cancer cells. Health gurus have been maintaining the colon health benefits of eating cabbage and sauerkraut for many years. The active component was called "cabbagen" before it was identified as a complex of indoles and isothiocyanates.

Cruciferous vegetables, garlic, and onions release their sulfur compounds when they are bruised, mashed, or cooked. In nature, one bite into green foods was enough to send many predators packing. For many adults, the strong taste of these vegetables has to be an acquired gustatory sensation. Nevertheless, the health benefits are well worth the effort.

About Spices and Culinary Herbs

The yellow and red spices and green culinary herbs listed in the first three food groups we are discussing are very high in antioxidants (carotenoids, sulfur, and polyphenols) and can contribute significant amounts to your daily total. Use them liberally and enjoy the excellent flavor they impart to your food while protecting your genes. A recent analysis of culinary herbs and spices has shown that the green herbs— oregano, marjoram, peppermint, rosemary, sage, tarragon, and thyme— contain the highest levels of antioxidants, followed by allspice, cinnamon, cloves, and saffron. Make sure to buy the highest-quality herbs and spices, and don't keep them in the cupboard too long. When the flavor begins to disappear, antioxidant levels drop.

Foods to Improve Gene Expression and Reset Genetic Switches

- *Colors:* purple, blue, black, magenta
- *Phytonutrients:* phenolics: flavonoids, polyphenols, anthocyanidins, plus vitamin C (a nonphenolic)
- *Serving size:* ½ cup
- *Servings per day:* 1–2

Fruit	Vegetables	Beverages	Spices (no limit)
Blackberries	Beets	Green and	All green leafy
Blueberries	Eggplant	black tea (3–4	herbs
Boysenberries	Radicchio	servings)	Allspice
Cherries		Juice from any of	Cardamom
Cranberries		the fruits listed	Cinnamon
Currants		Red wine	Curries
Grapes		White wine	Ginger
Marionberries			Peppermint
Pomegranates			
Prunes			
Raspberries			
Red apples			
Strawberries			

Note: During berry season, you can double up on purple fruits and choose yellow vegetables instead of a combination of yellow fruits and vegetables. Off-season, you can use frozen berries.

Why These Foods Are Important

Members of the berry, apple, and grape families make up this group of fruits. The diverse chemical structure of phenolic compounds determines their color, from colorless to deep purple or black. Phenolic compounds are a distinct class of water-soluble antioxidants that protect foods containing them from harsh weather. They protect proteins and DNA, for which they have a binding affinity. Thus, they help correct faulty genetic switching and improve protein expression.

Andreas Constantinou, Ph.D., is a well-known scientist from the University of Illinois–Chicago, specializing in cancer prevention. He made an important discovery in how two enzymes involved in DNA replication—DNA topiosomerase I and II—are activated. These enzymes cause breaks in one or both strands of DNA. Although these enzymes normally assist DNA replication, they can cause DNA damage as well. Amazingly, Dr. Constantinou and his team found that the phenolic compound ellagic acid inhibits these enzymes and thus prevents DNA damage. Perhaps the old adage, "An apple a day keeps the doctor away," really does apply.

More than 8,000 phenolic compounds are currently known, and they are natural antibiotics, anti-diarrheal, anti-ulcer, and anti-inflammatory agents. Foods rich in polyphenols are useful in the prevention or management of hypertension, vascular fragility, allergies, hypercholesterolemia, type 2 diabetes, and most other chronic diseases. Some phenolic compounds, such as those found in tea, bind to proteins including oral plaque, giving them unique anti-caries benefits.

Flavonoids are a large subgroup of phenolic compounds found in fruits, vegetables, whole grains, legumes, tea, and wine. Over 600 related compounds make up this family of powerful anti-aging nutrients. Large epidemiological studies have shown that flavonoids possess antioxidant, anti-inflammatory, and anti-thrombogenic properties. Additionally, some members of this family improve vascular function.

The ability of flavonoids to prevent heart attack was analyzed from data gathered in the Rotterdam study. This large study analyzed flavonoid intake among 4,807 men and women, with an average age of 67. The investigators found that drinking one to two cups of tea daily was protective against heart attack. Throughout the world, dietary flavonoids are consumed from wine, cranberry juice, grape juice, other berries and their juices, and less often from tea or cocoa, which is also a good source. Intake of berry juices, particularly cranberry, is tied to reduced risk of urinary tract infections.

Red wine contains a compound known as resveratrol, which scientists have found doubles the activity of a cellular anti-aging enzyme called sirtuin in species of worms and yeast. Moderate consumption of red wine may have a similar result in humans.

While berries and tea are some of the richest sources of flavonoids, apples and onions contain the highest levels of quercetin, an important flavonoid for fighting allergies. Lettuce and salad greens are also good sources of flavonoids but only if they are fresh and have been stored properly. Cut-up salad greens in bags have negligible flavonoid content, although they do contain other antioxidants. Eggplant contains the purple flavonoid glycoside nasunin, which is a potent scavenger of singlet oxygen-free radicals. Nasunin also sequesters iron, which reduces its pro-oxidant effects. Both of these functions are important protection against cardiovascular disease. Don't peel your eggplant!

The ability of flavonoids to inhibit aromatase, the enzyme responsible for estrogen dominance—a factor in some types of cancer—is an important consideration in anti-aging. Flavonoids also suppress the estrogenic activities of environmental estrogens (xenoestrogens) and thus help control estrogen dominance and estrogen-dependent cancers. Specifics on these effects will be discussed more fully in chapter 7.

Foods to Reduce Insulin Resistance and Balance Hormones

- *Colors:* tan, brown
- *Phytonutrients:* phytosterols, phytoestrogens, fiber, saponins, vitamin E, copper, zinc, magnesium, chromium
- *Serving size:* ½ cup
- *Servings per day:* 3–5

Breads Cereals, Grains	Rice, Pasta	Legumes	Vegetables	Nuts, Seeds
Barley	Amaranth	All beans	All potatoes	Almonds
Brown rice	Brown rice	Black-eyed	Brown mush-	Brazil nuts
Buckwheat	Couscous	peas	rooms	Cashews
Bulgur	Soba	Chickpeas	Edame	Filberts
Cornmeal	noodles	Lentils	(green	Flaxseeds
Millet	Tapioca	Miso paste	soybeans	Nut butters
Muesli	Whole-	Soy nuts	in pod)	Peanuts
Oat	grain	Split Peas	Green peas	Poppy seeds
Rye	pasta	Tempe		Sesame
Sorghum	Wild rice	Tofu		seeds
Triticale				Sunflower
Whole-				seeds
wheat				Walnuts
pita bread				

Why These Foods Are Important

Tan foods are carbohydrate-rich whole grains, legumes, and starchy vegetables. Nuts are included in this group because of the phytonutrients they contain, even though they contain oils and protein but very little carbohydrates. Tan foods are important sources of nutrients that are in short supply in our diet including dietary fiber, insoluble starches, trace minerals, B vitamins, vitamin E (tocopherols, tocotrienols), phytoestrogens, phytosterols, lignans, antioxidants, and polysaccharides with impressive anti-viral potential. Some of these foods contain phytoestrogens, which are powerful anti-cancer agents that help balance hormones. Phytosterols help reduce cholesterol. Several phytochemicals in whole tan foods are agents that block initial DNA damage and suppress carcinogenic processes.

Whole foods are also known to slow digestion and absorption of sugars. Investigators found that offering test subjects tan foods for breakfast improved satiety and reduced snacking and intake of food at the next meal. Furthermore, fiber-rich foods prevent insulin resistance and glycation of proteins. *Any process that disrupts the physical or botanical structure of food ingredients will increase blood glucose and insulin response.* Refined carbohydrates stripped of their phytonutrient components raise blood sugar too fast and drive us to eat bigger meals more frequently. Tan foods are very complex and contain a medicine chest of phytochemicals that retard aging and onset of aging conditions including cardiovascular disease, diabetes, and cancer.

Epidemiologists at Brigham and Women's Hospital in Boston analyzed data from 75,521 women and found a significant reduction in the incidence of stroke among those who ate the most whole grains and whole-grain products. They also concluded that a quick rise in blood sugar from eating refined carbohydrates raises the risk of cardiovascular disease regardless of other coronary disease risk factors that might be present.

Researchers at the University of Minnesota did a similar analysis of data on 35,988 Iowa women for the influence of carbohydrates on the development of type 2 diabetes. Intake of whole grains, fiber, and dietary magnesium offered protection against the development of this disease.

Dr. Edward Giovannucci's research team at Harvard gathered data from 43,757 male health professionals for 6 years. They found a significant reduction in coronary disease among the men with the highest intake of high-fiber cereal. The researchers also considered the benefits of fiber from fruit and vegetables, but these sources did not appear to be as protective. Soy protein has recently been promoted as particularly beneficial for the cardiovascular system, with claims to that effect now allowed by the Food and Drug Administration (FDA) on soy protein supplements.

How much soy protein should be consumed for cardiovascular benefits? Susan M. Potter, Ph.D., and colleagues from the University of Illinois, Urbana, wanted to answer this question. They replaced meat protein with soy protein in the diets of 81 men with mild hypercholesterolemia for 6 weeks. The men were divided into five groups, each receiving a different amount of soy protein. Surprisingly, those eating the smallest amount—20 grams, which is approximately 1 hefty scoop of soy protein powder per day—benefited as much as those who consumed larger amounts. Significant reductions in non-HDL cholesterol and apolipoprotein B—both risk factors for cardiovascular disease—were seen.

Legumes contain several disease-fighting phytochemicals including saponins, phytosterols, and isoflavones. Phytosterols inhibit intestinal cholesterol absorption, thereby lowering total cholesterol levels and LDL cholesterol. Among 590 people who participated in 16 separate clinical trials, phytosterol therapy reduced total cholesterol by 13 percent while LDL cholesterol dropped 30 percent.

Nuts have taken a bad rap for many years because they contain a high percentage of fat and sometimes salt. However, the fat is very good for you, and nuts contain a long list of beneficial phytonutrients. For example, almond skins contain nine different phenolic compounds with strong free radical–quenching capability. The phenolic compounds in walnuts protect LDL cholesterol from oxidation and thus help prevent atherosclerosis. New dietary guidelines from the American Heart Association's Dietary Approaches to Stop Hypertension (DASH) diet recommend several servings of nuts per week.

In addition to heart-friendly fats, nuts also contain protein, fiber, B vitamins, vitamins A and E, magnesium, calcium, copper, zinc, selenium, phosphorus, and potassium—and no cholesterol. Raw nuts are the best choice because most of these nutrients are located within the skin or just under it. Roasting—even dry roasting—destroys most of the benefits and adds unwanted fats, salt, and sugars.

Seeds also have significant health benefits. Flaxseed has long been favored as a bulking agent to improve bowel function. Recent evidence shows that adding flaxseeds to salads, cereals, and beverages improved blood lipid profiles. Flaxseeds also contain phytoestrogens called lignans that may help prevent bone loss among postmenopausal women.

Foods to Build DNA, Proteins, and Enzymes and Improve Intercellular Communication

- *Colors:* white, pale yellow, reddish brown (some)
- *Phytonutrients:* amino acids, essential fatty acids, vitamin A and other antioxidants (nuts, seeds, oils, eggs)
- *Serving size:* 1 ounce for proteins, 1 cup for dairy, 1 teaspoon for oils
- *Servings per day:* 8–14 ounces of protein, 2–3 dairy, 1–2 oils

Proteins	**Dairy**	**Oils**
Chicken	Kefir	Butter
Cottage cheese	Low-fat milk	Canola
Eggs	Soft cheese	Macadamia
Fish	Soy milk	Margarine
Legumes for vegetarians	Yogurt	Olive
Low-fat luncheon meats		Sesame
Low-fat or diet cheese		Salad dressings
Meat		
Organ meats		
Tofu		
Turkey		

Why These Foods Are Important

Protein foods to emphasize in your meal plans are those colored white. Although some fish are reddish in color, resulting from a carotenoid-rich diet, most are white fleshed. Fish contain healthy omega-3 oils, and fish consumption has been linked to reduction of several aging diseases including cardiovascular disease, cancer, and autoimmune conditions.

Red meat should be eaten infrequently, if at all. Wild game, buffalo, and ostrich are red meats that contain less saturated fat, are higher in zoochemicals (the animal equivalent of phytochemicals), and are easier to digest. Dairy products contain calcium and have been associated with reduced risk of colon cancer.

Eggs are an excellent source of fatty acids and vitamin A in addition to being high protein. If your diet is well balanced with lots of veggies and whole grains, the cholesterol in egg yolks should not be a problem. Eggs are highly digestible, and egg white is a nearly perfect protein. Some chickens are now being fed fish or algae meal, which makes their eggs an excellent source of docosahexaenoic acid (DHA). This fatty acid is concentrated in your brain and is essential for optimum cognitive function.

The popularity of high-protein diets for weight loss has caused scientists to rethink the ratios between carbohydrates, protein, and fats. For the first time, the U.S. Department of Agriculture is recommending an intake range. Newer guidelines suggest 20 to 30 percent of calories as protein, 30 percent as fat, and 40 to 50 percent as whole-grain carbohydrates.

It is important to increase protein intake as you age in order to maintain muscle mass, reduce insulin resistance, and repair DNA. However, excess intake of animal proteins makes the body more acidic, changing the cellular environment and making it less resistant to disease. Consequently, as animal protein intake increases, intake of fruits and vegetables that are alkaline must also increase to maintain optimal acid/base (pH) balance of the body. It's important to keep in mind that legumes and vegetables are excellent sources of protein as well. These sources do not alter pH balance and do not increase the rate of bone loss in postmenopausal women, in contrast to relying solely on animal proteins.

A general description of the benefits of healthy oils was already given. Here we emphasize the way oils overcome disease conditions. About 20 years ago, nutritionists were touting the health benefits of polyunsaturated oils. However, it was later discovered that these oils were easily oxidized inside the body, generating significant amounts of free radicals that damage DNA. A recent study by Scottish researchers found that when healthy subjects were fed a diet containing 5 to 15 percent of their total daily calories as polyunsaturated oils, their rate of DNA damage increased significantly. The damage was offset if the study participants took 80 milligrams of vitamin E (240 IU) daily. Eating natural-source oils from whole grains, fish, nut, and seed oils that come ready packaged with their own vitamin E is the best way you can fight aging.

Harvard scientists reviewed data from two large ongoing studies to determine the cardiovascular benefits of eating fish. Analysis of data from the male health professionals' study (43,671 men) revealed that eating fish just twice per month can reduce the risk of ischemic stroke and sudden death. Data from the nurses' health study (83,688 women) showed that eating fish from one to five times per week reduced risk of coronary heart disease between 20 and 33 percent. Greater benefit was found among those who ate the most fish. Another scientific team analyzing the nurses' data found that intake of omega-3 fatty acids (fish, walnuts, flaxseed oil) but not beta-carotene reduced risk of macular degeneration.

Vegetable oils also have significant health benefits. The typical Mediterranean diet that's high in monounsaturated fatty acids from olive oil has been found to protect against age-related cognitive decline. Olive oil appears to reduce the need for anti-hypertensive drugs by improving their utilization. The best olive oil is unrefined, dark green, extra-virgin oil. The color comes from naturally occurring antioxidants. Lighter oils may have had their antioxidants reduced by heating or bleaching during processing. And don't forget nut and seed oils.

From the Harvard Health Study, male professionals who ate nuts at least twice a week lowered their risk of sudden death by 47 percent and reduced their risk of coronary heart disease by 30 percent. Flaxseed oil, particularly with high lignan extraction, has significant hormone-balancing effects. It makes excellent salad dressing but is chemically unstable during cooking.

For great taste and cooking with high heat, the newest healthy oil is macadamia nut oil. This oil has a mild and pleasant taste, making it acceptable to those who don't like the strong taste of olive oil, and it can be used in baking. The vitamin E content of macadamia nut oil is four times that of olive oil, and it is extremely heat stable because of its high level of monounsaturated fatty acids.

Hidden and Dangerous Fats

Trans fats are ubiquitous in processed foods. They are considered one of the primary dietary promoters of cardiovascular disease. In 2003, the National Academy of Sciences recommended that the level of trans fats in the diet should be as low as possible. Amounts as low as 2 or 3 grams of trans fat a day can increase risk of heart disease. Look for hydrogenated or partially hydrogenated on food labels to identify those that contain trans fats. The nurses' health study revealed that women who ate the greatest amount of trans fats had a 50 percent greater risk of heart disease.

In July 2003, the Food and Drug Administration mandated that trans fats be listed on food and supplement labels by 2006. Reduce consumption of the following foods to cut back on trans fats (you don't have to eliminate them completely, just cut back):

Spreads
Margarine, stick
Mayonnaise
Salad dressings
Vegetable
    shortening

Fatty Proteins
American cheese
Frankfurters
Luncheon meats
Sausage

Snacks
Cheese crackers
Frozen desserts
Ice cream
Microwave
    popcorn
Milkshakes
Potato and tortilla
    chips
Salted crackers

Fried Foods
Deep fried onion
    rings or chicken
    nuggets

Baked Goods
(prepared)
Biscuit mix
Bread crumbs
Cake mixes
Canned frostings
Chocolate candy bars
Cookies
Corn muffin mix
Danish pastry
Dinner rolls
Dough, refrigerated
Hamburger buns
Pound cake
Sweet rolls

Doughnuts   Taco shells
French fries   White bread

Note: Butter and soft tub margarine do not contain trans fats and are the preferred
spreads.

Special Considerations

Although the color of food reveals its phytonutrient content, it does
not tell you which foods contain the most natural sugars. Since we get
more insulin resistant as we grow older, it is important to know how
quickly foods are turned into glucose. As you have already learned, the
closer a food is to its natural state, the better balanced it is. For example, fruit is high in natural sugars. Yet the fiber in whole fruit helps slow
the processing of its sugars into glucose. In contrast, fruit juice does not
contain much fiber and is quickly converted into glucose. You can also
slow down the conversion of fruit sugars into glucose by eating protein
foods first. However, eating fruit with proteins gives many people indigestion. Vegetable juices, with the exception of carrot juice, are more
slowly converted into glucose because they contain protein and are a
better choice with meals.

The measure of how quickly a food is digested into glucose is called
the glycemic index. Low-glycemic foods include

All-bran cereals	Grapefruit	Peanuts
Apple juice	Grapes	Pears
Apples	Ice cream	Peas
Barley	(in moderation)	Plums
Berries	Milk	Soybeans
Black-eyed peas	Muesli cereal	Strawberries
Bulgur	Navy beans	Wild rice
Butter beans	Oranges	Yogurt (no added
Cherries	Peaches	sugar)

Moderate-glycemic foods that are commonly found in the American diet are not necessarily the healthiest choices. Nevertheless, you
can enjoy them in moderation. They include

Basmati rice	Potato chips
Beets	Potatoes (red, white)
Buckwheat	Pumpernickel bread
Carrots	Raisins

Cereal (low sugar)   Sourdough bread
Corn on the cob   Spaghetti
Lima beans   Sucrose (table sugar)
Oatmeal   Sweet potatoes
Pasta   Whole-wheat bread (100% stone ground)
Peas

High-glycemic foods can be enjoyed by most people but may not be well tolerated by those with severe blood sugar problems. They include

Apricots   Mangoes
Bagels   Muffins
Bananas (ripe)   Pancakes
Breakfast cereals (refined with   Papayas
  added sugar)   Parsnips
Corn chips   Potatoes (baked)
Corn flakes   Puffed rice or wheat
Corn syrup solids   Rice cakes
Crackers   Shredded wheat
Doughnuts   Soft drinks and sport drinks
Glucose and glucose polymers   (added sugars)
  (maltodextrin)   Toaster waffles
Hamburger and hot dog buns   Watermelon
Honey   White bread
Jelly beans   White rice
Maltose   Whole-wheat bread

Although some foods on this list contain healthy phytonutrients, they should not make up your daily meal plans. Eating several foods on this list frequently and on the same day increases your body's demand for insulin. Apricots, papayas, mangoes, and watermelon are so high in carotenes that you should enjoy them when in season. Avoid frequent consumption of canned or dried apricots.

Diet and Pain

Many aging conditions cause pain, and diet affects pain intensity. You'll find that phytochemicals in certain groups of foods—solanaceae or nightshades, for example—can exacerbate joint pain. Potatoes, tomatoes, bell peppers, and eggplant are members of this family. Wine and aged cheeses contain tyramines that elevate monoamine oxidase, reduce serotonin, and cause pain in susceptible individuals. Aspartame (e.g., Equal®) contains phenylalanine, which can further reduce serotonin. Monosodium glutamate (MSG) is a popular flavor enhancer, especially in Asian dishes, but is also a powerful neurochemical that causes pain in some people. Some foods such as nuts and citrus are healthy foods but are common allergens. Foods that may cause pain include

Aged cheese	Coffee	Solanaceae (arthritis)
Alcohol	Dairy products	Sugar
Aspartame	Margarine	Tea
Caffeine products	Meat	Wheat
Carbonated beverages	MSG	White flour
Citrus	Nuts	Wine

Healing foods are listed in our menus and are well tolerated by most. Some, such as fish and seed oils, are also suggested as dietary supplements to ease pain. Foods that fight pain include

Alaska salmon; yellowfin, bigeye, or albacore tuna; herring; anchovies; sardines; mackerel; lake trout	Flaxseed, canola, and walnut oils
	Fruit (except citrus)
	Legumes
	Red, yellow, orange, and green
Barley, oats, millet	vegetables
Brown rice	Spelt, teff, quinoa
Dark leafy greens	

We will offer suggestions of dietary supplements that help reduce inflammation and fight pain in chapter 6. Now that we have completed our discussion of the science behind a good diet, it's time to plan our menus.

Implementing the Anti-Aging Eating Plan

Anti-aging eating will give you the basic platform for taking charge of your aging. The basic meal plan is the same for everyone, with serving sizes adjusted for ideal weights. You may need to consider certain foods in planning meals in order to reduce certain conditions. For example, if you are diabetic, you will do best if you concentrate on low-glycemic foods and avoid those that quickly turn into glucose when you eat them. If you suffer from chronic pain, you will need to focus on foods that relieve pain and avoid those that cause pain.

Let's begin with an honest evaluation of the foods and beverages you are now consuming. Most people aren't sure how much of each food they actually eat. Therefore, we suggest you keep a diary for a few days to check what you're eating. You will find a nutrition quiz in appendix B.

The first step in following the anti-aging meal plans is to determine which serving sizes you should consume. Five levels of servings are offered, and each corresponds to a specific weight category and exercise level for women and men. For those over 50, we have provided a third category, and the recommendations for men and women in this category are the same. You will note that the meal plans provide for a maximum of 2,600 calories per day. Scientists agree that keeping caloric intake moderate is the only proven way to extend life, as we discussed earlier in this chapter.

To use the meal planner conversion chart, you should

1. Find which of the categories applies to you: female, male, or either gender over 51 years old
2. Find the correct column for your activity level based on the number of hours of exercise you do each week
3. Find the row that represents your present weight or optimum weight if you need to lose some weight

MEAL PLANNER CONVERSION CHART

Women (25–50 years)	Activity Level	
	Low to Medium	Medium to High
	0–4 hours of exercise per week	5–10 hours of exercise per week
Weight 110–140 pounds (50–62 kg)	Group B (1,800 calories)	Group C (2,200 calories)
Weight 141–180 pounds (63–82 kg)	Group C (2,200 calories)	Group D (2,400 calories)

Men (25–50 years)	Activity Level	
	Low to Medium	Medium to High
	0–4 hours of exercise per week	5–10 hours of exercise per week
Weight under 155 pounds (70 kg)	Group C (2,200 calories)	Group D (2,400 calories)

Weight 155–180 pounds	Group D	Group E
(71–82 kg)	(2,400 calories)	(2,600 calories)

Women and Men	Activity Level	
(51 + years)		
	Low to Medium	Medium to High
	0–4 hours of exercise per week	5–10 hours of exercise per week
Weight 110–140 pounds (50–62 kg)	Group A (1,500 calories)	Group B (1,800 calories)
Weight 141–180 pounds (63–82 kg)	Group B (1,800 calories)	Group C (2,200 calories)

Note: If you are a competitive athlete or are very active, choose the next higher meal planner category (e.g., C instead of B) or add one additional meal per day.

Now that you have studied the meal planner conversion chart, it's time to implement your plan step by step.

Step 1: Circle the correct group letter. You will use this group letter to identify your daily menu plans later in this chapter. My meal planner category is

1. Group A
2. Group B
3. Group C
4. Group D
5. Group E

Step 2: All groups should follow these guidelines in planning daily menus:

1. Plan two protein-based meals featuring eggs, lunch meat, fish, poultry, beans, dairy, or cheese.
2. Plan one tan starch–based meal featuring cereal, breads, pasta, starchy vegetable, or rice.
3. Alternate meals so that you follow a carbohydrate meal with one high in protein. You will notice that breakfast features fruit and fruit or vegetable juice. These items can also be reserved for later in the day as snacks.

4. Make vegetables a main part of lunch and dinner, regardless of whether the meal is protein or carbohydrate based. Vegetables may also be part of breakfast. For example, a vegetable omelet can contain 1 or 2 servings of veggies. Cook extra veggies for dinner, then use them for breakfast or other meals the following day. Tuck greens into sandwiches and use raw veggies as snacks. Look for ways to add veggies to everything you eat and it becomes easy to achieve your optimum servings of these anti-aging foods.

Plan one large or two smaller salads each day. In addition, eat 1 cup of steamed veggies. Or, you may wish to make a large salad your main meal and add 3 to 4 protein servings (shrimp, cottage cheese, beans, chicken). Here's how you should think about salads: A small salad served on a 6-inch plate with greens and raw veggies of your choice, containing 2 cups greens, ½ cup raw veggies (¼ cup if cooked), equals 3 servings. A medium salad served on a 7-inch plate, containing 3 cups greens and 1 cup raw veggies, equals 4 servings. A large salad served on a 9-inch plate, containing 4 cups greens and 1 to 2 cups raw veggies, equals 5 to 6 servings.

What if you just can't handle a lot of raw veggies? Will you be compromising nutrition to subdue them with cooking? Some enzyme activity is lost when vegetables are steamed, but many nutrients are more bioavailable when vegetables are cooked. For example, carotenoids are released when cooking breaks down the cellulose matrix that traps them. For centuries, ancient healers have advised patients to eat steamed veggies because they are more digestible. Keep in mind that cooking reduces the volume of veggies you have to eat. A 1-pound bag of baby spinach when steamed makes only 2 cups or 4 servings—lots easier to swallow!

The important thing is to make sure the vegetables are not over-cooked. We suggest purchasing an electric steamer with a timer for cooking veggies. You can also cook them quickly in a wok. The veggies render a nice juice that makes them ideal companions for tossing with pasta. Add a handful of fresh herbs and you have an elegant meal.

Another helpful tip is to put 1 cup of raw greens with something hot so that the greens wilt. For example, put spinach or arugula in the middle of an omelet or under a chop, fish fillet, or other protein. It adds wonderful flavor and gets in another veggie serving. In cooler weather, wilted greens make wonderful salads. Suggested wilted green salads are given in this chapter.

There are five food groups plus oils to keep track of in planning your daily meals. We begin the detailed menu plans with vegetables because they present the greatest challenge for most people. Yet they are the key to improving health and longevity.

Daily Menu Plans for Group A

This group includes physically inactive people over 51 years old weighing 140 pounds or less and those who want to lose weight.

Veggies: Seven ½-cup servings of cooked veggies; 1cup raw as in salads. Note: Each vegetable serving contains ¼ serving of protein.

Note that the servings calculated for these salads are based on raw veggies. If you use cooked veggies, you can cut the cups listed in half.

Fruit: 2 fruits. Eat 1 medium-size yellow/orange fruit or 1 cup of berries plus a glass of juice. Keep in mind it's better to eat fruits and skip the juice, since juice is higher in natural sugar. Berries, fresh or frozen, and berry or grape juice are available year-round, so you should make sure to include them in your daily meal plans. If you choose veggie juice (V-8 or carrot), you may wish to use fruit on top of cottage cheese or in place of veggies on one of your salads. When making fruit salads, subtract a corresponding number of fruit servings from your breakfast the next day.

Proteins: 8 ounces of lean or low-fat items divided into two meals. Proteins are relatively easier to work with. You can choose eggs for breakfast, and fish, poultry, or meat for one other meal. You can also eat a cottage cheese (½ cup is a protein serving) salad plus another protein for one other meal. Beans, split peas, or lentils (½ cup is a protein serving) make an excellent choice for a protein meal.

Tan starchy foods: Four ½-cup servings. This may seem like very little, but keep in mind that you are getting additional carbohydrates in your fruit and veggies. Most people eat too many white starchy foods that are devoid of nutrients other than calories. As you have seen, a diet high in these foods can lead to serious problems involving insulin resistance.

Choose whole-grain sugar-free cereals; multigrain bagels, English muffins, or waffles; or any whole-grain tan food on carbo-based breakfast days. You can add a slice of bread for lunch if you have a protein-based breakfast, or have rice or pasta for dinner if you don't have bread for lunch. Limit tan food selections to just one or two meals per day.

Dairy: Two 1-cup low-fat selections. Have one of these servings for breakfast and the other before bedtime or as a snack during the day.

Oils: 1 teaspoon of whipped butter or soft tub margarine and 2 tablespoons of oil for cooking or salads, or 2 tablespoons of mayonnaise instead of butter as a spread. Using low-fat salad dressings, spreads, and cooking spray dramatically cuts down on your fat intake. Fat-free items are not good choices because various sugars have been substituted for fats. Try nut butters (tan foods) as spreads on toast or whole-grain bread products.

Key: ounce—oz.; cup—c.; teaspoon—t.; tablespoon—T.

SUGGESTED 4-DAY MENU PLAN FOR GROUP A

Breakfast	Protein Based	Carbo Based	Carbo Based	Protein Based
	2-egg or 3-egg-white omelet 1 fruit 6 oz. orange juice 8 oz. hot chocolate	1 c. cereal ¾ c. milk 1 fruit 6 oz. V-8 or carrot juice	4-inch-square waffle 1 t. butter 1 c. strawberries 1 c. yogurt 6 oz. cranberry juice	Shake containing 16 grams protein from whey or soy protein powder made with 1 c. yogurt, 6 oz. orange juice, 1 mashed banana, 1 T. wheat germ or flaxseeds

Lunch	Carbo Based	Protein Based	Protein Based	Protein Based
	Pasta and veggie sauce: 1 c. pasta, ½ c. veggies left over from dinner Small salad 1 T. low-fat dressing	4 oz. turkey on 1 slice whole-grain bread 1 T. mayo 3 tomato slices 1 c. raw broccoli, carrots, celery, etc. Low-fat dip	4 oz. chicken cut up on medium salad ¼ c. sunflower seeds Balsamic vinegar or lemon juice	Medium salad with 1 sliced hard-boiled egg and 4 oz. shrimp Lemon juice or 1 T. low-fat dressing

Dinner	Protein Based	Protein Based	Protein Based	Carbo Based
	7 oz. steamed salmon Small salad	4 oz. lean steak 1 medium ear corn on the	4 oz. grilled halibut ½ c. veggies	1½ c. pasta tossed with 1½ c. veggies

½ c. steamed veggies 1 T. low-fat dressing	cob 1 t. butter Medium salad Balsamic vinegar	Small salad 1 T. low-fat dressing	One 2-oz. meat-ball Small salad 1 T. olive oil and 1 T. lemon juice

Bedtime

8 oz. milk	8 oz. yogurt with fruit	8 oz. kefir	8 oz. soymilk

Daily Menu Plans for Group B

This group includes physically inactive people 25 to 50 years old weighing 140 pounds or less and those wanting to lose weight.

Veggies: Ten ½-cup servings (or 1 cup if raw). Plan on eating one large or two smaller salads containing 2 to 4 cups of greens topped with ½ to ¾ cup of raw veggies. In addition, have 1½ cups of steamed veggies for dinner. You can make your main meal of the day a large salad with lots of veggies. Add some beans or other protein to make it a high-protein meal.

Fruit: 2 fruits—1 yellow and 1 purple.

Proteins: 10 ounces. Plan two protein-centered meals each day.

Tan starchy foods: Five ½-cup servings. Plan only one tan starchy-centered meal a day. A second serving, say crackers or a slice of bread, may accompany another meal that is high protein.

Dairy: Two 1-cup low-fat selections.

Oils: 1 teaspoon of whipped butter or soft tub margarine and 2 tablespoons of oil.

SUGGESTED 4-DAY MENU PLAN FOR GROUP B

Breakfast	Protein Based	Carbo Based	Carbo Based	Protein Based
	2-egg or 3-egg-white omelet with ½ c. cooked veggies 1 fruit 6 oz. orange juice	1½ c. cereal 1 c. milk 2 fruits 6 oz. V-8 or carrot juice	Two 4-inch-square waffles 1 t. butter 1 c. strawberries 1 c. yogurt 6 oz. cranberry juice	Shake containing 16 grams protein from whey or soy protein powder made with 1 c. yogurt, 6 oz. orange juice,

8 oz. hot chocolate 1 slice whole-grain toast with 1 T. peanut butter			1 mashed banana, 1 T. wheat germ or flaxseeds

Lunch	Carbo Based	Protein Based	Protein Based	Protein Based
	Pasta and veggie sauce: 2 c. pasta, 1½ c. veggies left over from dinner One 2-oz. meatball left over from dinner Small salad 1 T. low-fat dressing	4 oz. turkey on 1 slice whole-grain bread 1 T. mayo 3 tomato slices ½ c. lettuce 1½ c. raw broccoli, carrots, celery, etc. Low-fat dip	4 oz. chicken cut up on medium salad ¼ c. sunflower seeds Balsamic vinegar or lemon juice	Medium salad with 1 sliced hard-boiled egg and 4 oz. shrimp Lemon juice or 1 T. low-fat dressing 4 small crackers

Dinner	Protein Based	Protein Based	Protein Based	Carbo Based
	7 oz. steamed salmon Small salad 1 c. steamed veggies 1 T. low-fat dressing	6 oz. lean steak 2 medium ears corn on the cob 1 t. butter Small salad ¼ c. croutons Balsamic vinegar	6 oz. grilled halibut 1½ c. veggies Small salad 1 T. low-fat dressing 1½ c. brown rice	2 c. pasta with 1½ c. veggies Two 2-oz. meatballs Medium salad 1 T. olive oil and 1 T. lemon juice

Bedtime				
	8 oz. milk	8 oz. yogurt with fruit	8 oz. kefir	8 oz. soymilk

Menu plans A and B will satisfy most people past middle age. If you are a large person or physically very active, you may need one of the following plans. You'll notice that the additional calories come largely from vegetables and protein, although all of the plans contain the same percentages of protein, carbohydrates, and fats.

Daily Menu Plans for Group C

This group includes physically active people over 51 years old weighing 141 pounds or more; physically active women 25 to 50 years old weighing 140 pounds or less; physically inactive women 25 to 50 weighing 141 pounds or more; physically inactive men 25 to 50 weighing 155 pounds or more.

If you fit into the third category listed above and you are overweight or have a high BMI, you should consider following the menu plans for either group A or B in order to promote longevity. Exercise plans in chapter 5 will also help you lose weight and live longer.

Veggies: Twelve ½-cup servings.

Fruit: 3 fruits.

Proteins: 12 ounces.

Tan starchy foods: Six ½-cup servings.

Dairy: Two 1-cup servings.

Oils: 1½ teaspoons of whipped butter or soft tub margarine and 3 tablespoons of oil.

SUGGESTED 4-DAY MENU PLAN FOR GROUP C

Breakfast	Protein Based	Carbo Based	Carbo Based	Protein Based
	3-egg or 4-egg-white omelet with 1½ c. veggies 2 fruits 6 oz. orange juice 12 oz. hot chocolate 1 slice whole-grain toast with 2 T. almond butter	2 c. cereal 1½ c. milk 2 fruits 6 oz. V-8 or carrot juice	Two 4-inch-square waffles 1½ t. butter 1 c. strawberries 1½ c. yogurt 6 oz. cranberry juice 1 c. melon or orange pieces	Shake containing 24 grams protein from whey or soy protein powder with 1½ c. yogurt, 6 oz. orange juice, 1 mashed banana, 1 T. wheat germ or flaxseeds

Lunch	Carbo Based	Protein Based	Protein Based	Protein Based
	Pasta and veggie sauce: 2 c. pasta, 2 c.	4 oz. turkey on 1 slice whole-grain bread	4 oz. chicken cut up on medium salad	Medium salad with 1 sliced hard-boiled

veggies left over from dinner	½ c. lettuce	¼ c. sunflower seeds	egg and 5 oz. shrimp
One 2-oz. meatball left over from dinner	3 tomato slices	¼ c. croutons	Lemon juice or
	2 T. mayo	Balsamic vinegar	1 T. low-fat
	1½ c. raw broccoli, carrots,	or lemon juice	dressing
Small salad	celery, etc.		4 small crackers
1 T. low-fat dressing	Low-fat dip		

Dinner	Protein Based	Protein Based	Protein Based	Carbo Based
	9 oz. steamed salmon	8 oz. lean steak	8 oz. grilled halibut	2½ c. pasta with 2 c. veggies
	Medium salad	2 medium ears corn on the cob	2 c. veggies	Two 2-oz. meatballs
	1½ c. steamed veggies	1 t. butter	Medium salad	Medium salad
	1½ c. brown rice	Medium salad	1 T. low-fat dressing	1 T. olive oil and 1 T. lemon juice
		¼ c. croutons	1½ c. brown rice	
		1 T. low-fat dressing		

Bedtime				
	8 oz. milk	8 oz. yogurt with fruit	8 oz. kefir	8 oz. soymilk

Daily Menu Plans for Group D

This group includes physically active women ages 25 to 50 weighing more than 140 pounds; physically active men ages 25 to 50 weighing less than 155 pounds; physically inactive men ages 25 to 50 weighing 155 pounds or more.

If you find yourself in this group and are not physically active, you should consider either plan B or plan C. You may need to lower your BMI in order to avoid the aging pitfalls of being overweight. The exercise suggestions in chapter 5 will also help you achieve a more favorable body composition. If you are active, study the suggestions in chapter 5 to make sure you are not sabotaging your anti-aging goals by overtraining or not getting enough antioxidants.

Veggies: Thirteen ½-cup servings.

Fruit: 3 fruits.

Proteins: 13 ounces.

Tan starchy foods: Seven ½-cup servings.

Dairy: Three 1-cup servings.

Oils: 2 teaspoons of whipped butter or soft tub margarine and 4 tablespoons of oil.

SUGGESTED 4-DAY MENU PLAN FOR GROUP D

Breakfast	Protein Based	Carbo Based	Carbo Based	Protein Based
	3-egg or 4-egg-white omelet with 1½ c. veggies 2 fruits 6 oz. orange juice 12 oz. hot chocolate 1 slice whole-grain toast with 2 T. almond butter	2 c. cereal 1½ c. milk 2 fruits 12 oz. V-8 or carrot juice	Two 4-inch-square waffles 1½ t. butter 1 c. strawberries 1½ c. yogurt 6 oz. cranberry juice 1 c. melon or orange pieces	Shake containing 24 grams protein from whey or soy protein powder, 1½ c. yogurt, 12 oz. orange juice, 1 mashed banana, 1 T. wheat germ or flaxseeds

Lunch	Carbo Based	Protein Based	Protein Based	Protein Based
	Pasta and veggie sauce: 2 c. pasta, 1½ c. veggies left over from dinner One 2-oz. meatball left over from dinner Medium salad 2 T. low-fat dressing	5 oz. turkey on 2 slices whole-grain bread ½ c. lettuce 4 tomato slices 2 T. mayo 1½ c. raw broccoli, carrots, celery, etc. Low-fat dip Small bunch of grapes	5 oz. chicken cut up on medium salad ¼ c. sunflower seeds ¼ c. croutons Balsamic vinegar or lemon juice	Large salad with 1 sliced hard-boiled egg and 6 oz. shrimp Lemon juice or 2 T. low-fat dressing 5 small crackers

Dinner	Protein Based	Protein Based	Protein Based	Carbo Based
	11 oz. steamed salmon	8 oz. lean steak 2 medium ears	8 oz. grilled halibut	2½ c. pasta with 2½ c. veggies

Medium salad	corn on the	2 c. veggies	Two 2-oz. meat-
1½ c. steamed	cob	Medium salad	balls
veggies	1 t. butter	1½ c. brown rice	Large salad
1½ c. brown rice	Medium salad	1 T. low-fat	2 T. olive oil
	¼ c. croutons	dressing	and 2 T. lemon
	Low-fat dressing		juice

Bedtime

12 oz. milk	12 oz. yogurt with fruit	12 oz. kefir	12 oz. soymilk

Daily Menu Plans for Group E

This group includes very physically active men ages 25 to 50 weighing 155 pounds or more.

These menu plans are intended for men whose work is physically demanding or who are serious athletes. Those who are competitive athletes can also use this plan but depending upon the sport may need to increase servings to achieve daily caloric needs. If you are in this category, be sure to maintain the same ratio between food groups, increasing vegetable and fruit intake as well as proteins and carbohydrates. You can easily do this by adding servings from one of the lower-calorie groups such as Group B (1,800 calories) or Group C (2,200 calories).

Veggies: Fourteen ½-cup servings.

Fruit: 3 fruits.

Proteins: 14 ounces.

Tan starchy foods: Seven ½-cup servings.

Dairy: Three 1-cup servings.

Oils: 2 teaspoons of whipped butter or soft tub margarine and 4 tablespoons of oil.

SUGGESTED 4-DAY MENU PLAN FOR GROUP E

Breakfast	Protein Based	Carbo Based	Carbo Based	Protein Based
	3-egg or 4-egg-white omelet with 2 c. cooked veggies	2 c. cereal 1½ c. milk 2 fruits 12 oz. V-8 or carrot juice	Two 4-inch-square waffles 2 t. butter 1 c. strawberries 1½ c. yogurt	Shake containing 32 grams protein from whey or soy protein powder

	2 fruits 6 oz. orange juice 12 oz. hot chocolate 1 slice whole-grain toast with 2 T. almond butter		6 oz. cranberry juice 1 c. melon or orange pieces	with 1½ c. yogurt, 12 oz. orange juice, 1 mashed banana, 1 T. wheat germ or flaxseeds

	Carbo Based	Protein Based	Protein Based	Protein Based
Lunch	Pasta and veggie sauce: 2 c. pasta, left over from dinner 2 c. veggies Two 2-oz. meatballs left over from dinner Large salad with 2 T. low-fat dressing	6 oz. turkey on 2 slices whole-grain bread ½ c. lettuce 4 tomato slices 2 T. mayo 2 c. raw broccoli, carrots, celery, etc. Low-fat dip Small bunch of grapes	6 oz. chicken cut up on medium salad ¼ c. sunflower seeds ¼ c. croutons Balsamic vinegar or lemon juice	Làrge salad with 1 sliced hard-boiled egg and 8 oz. shrimp Lemon juice or 2 T. low-fat dressing 6 small crackers

	Protein Based	Protein Based	Protein Based	Carbo Based
Dinner	10 oz. steamed salmon Medium salad 1½ c. steamed veggies 1½ c. brown rice	8 oz. lean steak 2 medium ears corn on the cob 1 t. butter Medium salad ¼ c. croutons Low-fat dressing	8 oz. grilled halibut 2 c. veggies Medium salad 1½ c. brown rice 1 T. low-fat dressing	3 c. pasta with 2½ c. veggies Three 2-oz. meatballs Large salad 2 T. olive oil and 2 T. lemon juice

Bedtime	12 oz. milk	12 oz. yogurt with fruit	12 oz. kefir	12 oz. soymilk

Suggested Salad Combinations

Salads can be varied, adding an element of color and interest to any meal. These are some combinations you may want to try. They are fun and creative and will require some adjustment in servings of the food groups in your daily plans. Most of these salads are combinations of veggies and fruit that will eliminate a fruit serving from breakfast. Many also contain seeds that reduce the servings of tan starchy foods you'll need.

Sprouts are a wonderful addition to any salad or sandwich. Choose mung, aduki, red clover, black radish, alfalfa, pea, sunflower, and broccoli. You can sprout any of these from seeds in your kitchen using a sprouter.

Dress the salads with balsamic vinegar or lemon juice and macadamia nut, flax, grapeseed, or olive oil. You can also use low-fat dressings. Avoid fat-free dressings because they are generally high in sugars. Here are some suggestions:

- Radicchio topped with orange slices, pecans, and feta cheese
- Arugula topped with grated baby turnips, blood oranges, and tamari sunflower seeds
- Baby spinach topped with sliced pears, avocados, and poppy seeds
- Romaine lettuce topped with cucumber slices, grated daikon radish or jicama, and pine nuts
- Endive topped with tangerine sections, pimento or roasted red peppers, and walnuts
- Mixed baby greens topped with shredded apple, radish, celery, and sliced almonds
- Chopped cabbage topped with shredded carrots, asparagus, and sesame seeds
- Frisee topped with grapefruit sections, mangoes, and pomegranate seeds
- Endive and baby bok choy topped with sliced kiwi fruit, papaya or pineapple, and toasted soy nuts
- Spinach prepared with a warm bacon dressing, celery seed, hard-boiled eggs, roasted red peppers, and croutons

You can choose mixes of kale, baby chard, baby beet tops, turnip greens, collards, and mustard greens for braising. It's important to get very young, tender leaves. Sauté them with garlic, onions or leeks, and butternut squash. Toss them with pasta or rice for a complete meal. You can also add bite-size pieces of chicken, tuna, or pork.

Ideas for Fish

Fish contain omega-3 fatty acids that promote cardiovascular health and are anti-inflammatory and anti-tumor. We recommend 2 or 3 servings of fish per week, choosing among salmon, trout, sole, halibut, catfish, snapper, and shellfish. These fish feed on vegetation and are less likely to contain mercury. Limit your intake of large predator fish such as tuna, shark, swordfish, and large bass species, even though scientists are questioning the concern over mercury. The form of mercury in seafood differs from that used in toxicology tests and may not present the risk for women of child-bearing age that was previously thought.

Fish are quick and easy to prepare by steaming, baking, stewing, or adding to stir-fried vegetables. Here are some suggestions:

- Steamed salmon fillets topped with fresh dill, capers, and served on a bed of radicchio or chicory
- Steamed salmon steaks topped with spicy vegetable low-fat cheese or roasted peppers and low-fat cream cheese
- Grilled halibut topped with mango salsa
- Baked fillets of sole topped with lemon slices, capers, and white wine
- Macadamia nut–encrusted baked cod

Converting Nutrition Information into Food Groups

You will want to expand your menu plans to include soups and combination dishes. Look for recipes that contain nutrition information, then you can make the following substitutions in your daily meal plan. You will have to decide whether the dish is primarily protein or carbohydrate based and the amount of vegetables. For example, protein will be pretty straightforward, although some will come from vegetables and starches. Carbohydrates are a little trickier. You'll have to decide which food category the dish fits best. Combination dishes can be high in fat. Keep in mind that oils are healthier than saturated fats, and you can usually cut down on the fat called for in a recipe by substituting low-fat alternatives. This is obviously not an exact science because foods are complex, containing various amounts of proteins, carbohydrates, and oils, but it's a convenient method to use. You can find dairy servings listed among recipe ingredients. Their protein, carbohydrate, and fat contents will be contained in the nutrition information.

- *Proteins:* 7 grams of protein = 1 protein serving
- *Vegetables:* 5 grams of carbohydrates = 1 vegetable serving
- *Fruit:* 15 grams of carbohydrates = 1 fruit serving
- *Tan starchy foods:* 15 grams of carbohydrates = 1 tan serving
- *Fats:* 5 grams of fat = 1 serving

Bon appétit!

CHAPTER 5

Step 3: Exercise Your Genes

The joy of life consists in the exercise of one's energies, continual growth, constant change, the enjoyment of every new experience. To stop means simply to die.

—Aleister Crowley

The Anti-Aging Workout

An integral part of the anti-aging solution is fitness. Anti-aging exercises help mold your body into more youthful contours, reduce stress, and balance hormones. Exercise even determines what foods you'll choose at your next meal. And, of course, the weight-loss benefits of exercise are well known. We have to make a serious effort to fit exercise into the daily life of our genes because modern lifestyle provides too much psychological stress and not enough physical exertion.

Before the 1950s, Americans didn't have to worry much about getting enough exercise. People walked or rode bicycles to work. Many worked long hours on farms or in factories. People living in cities didn't even own a car, while those in the suburbs had one family car. Parents didn't drive their children around. Kids walked, biked, or rode a bus, and they had a routine list of chores that had to be done to keep family life running smoothly.

Work around the home was more exercise intensive because fewer gadgets designed for easy living were available. Convenience foods were unheard of and eating out was reserved for special occasions.

Today, with hundreds of time-saving conveniences, we find we're too tired and too busy to feed ourselves properly! Many people work in front of a computer all day, grab something quick to satiate hunger, then go home and watch TV until bedtime. Consequently, we have become a fat and unfit nation. Our lack of exercise is killing us!

We have to plan our exercise now, whereas it used to be part of everyday activities. The anti-aging workout plan offers practical tips on adding exercise to your daily routine without worrying about making it to the gym. To help reach anti-aging goals, your workout makeover brings fitness into everything you do.

As we grow older, our stamina, strength, balance, coordination, and flexibility are all reduced. It happens gradually and we don't realize it. While we lose physical strength and stamina as we age, hopefully we do gain some wisdom. So, don't beat yourself up because you can't keep the same pace you did when you were in your twenties. Change your exercise goals. Although it may be trendy to say you work out, it may not be possible to have washboard abs. You need to work smarter and think about exercise in a different way. Here is Carol's story, which will resonate with many of you who are exercising to prevent aging:

> I have always been a physical person, although I wouldn't say I'm really athletic. Yet I have pushed myself to compete in swimming, hiking, and biking. Although I am now in my early fifties, I have cut myself little slack since in many ways I feel younger than I did at twenty. I swim several times a week, lift weights, and speed walk. I also eat well and have meditated for many years to counter stress levels.
>
> Consequently, it came as a surprise to me that I had lost considerable range of motion and balance—something I learned through a cycling accident. While riding down a steep grade on my mountain bike, I was unable to avoid hitting a large rock that was partly buried in tall grass and I took a nasty spill. I was able to collect myself and my bike and head home, but after a few hours I realized that something was seriously wrong with my knee. A trip to the doctor confirmed my suspicions; I had cracked the head of my lower leg bone and strained a couple of ligaments. I was now on crutches and faced with months of therapy. The therapy I undertook taught me to think smarter about how I work my body, and it has made a huge difference in the benefits I gain from exercise. I began with a flotation device and

movement in the water. In 1 month, I began working with a Pilates trainer who specialized in physical therapy.

Gradually, I came to realize that working smarter means building strength, balance, and range of motion through a wide range of exercises. I was working muscles that I hadn't accessed through the weight circuit. Instead of powering through exercises, I learned how much more effectively the body functions when careful attention is paid to how various muscle groups are being worked. I got the same "high" from my workouts without the pain—just lots of muscle awareness. What surprised me the most was how toned and fit my body became. I have gained about 7 pounds in weight, but it's muscle. My waist is now a couple of inches smaller and I have a flatter stomach and better hip profile. I now realize that had I been exercising smarter, I probably wouldn't have crashed and burned on my bike.

The physiological effects of meditation have only recently begun to be studied. Researchers have shown that long-term practice of meditation improves oxygenation of tissues, heart rhythm, and brain function. In chapter 3, we discussed how meditation affects hormone and neurotransmitter function. Here we mention meditation again because it supports many of the goals of our anti-aging exercise plan.

Benefits of Movement Exercise

	Benefits	**Type of Exercise**
Movement exercises	Improved balance and flexibility	Tai chi
	Brain stimulation (improved hormonal stimulation)	Qi gong
	Improved posture	Soft martial arts
	Improved sleep	Dance
	Cardio fitness	

Tai chi and qi gong are meditative exercises that have been practiced in Asia for centuries. The first impression most Westerners have is that the slow rhythmic movements of tai chi hardly qualify as exercise. Yet the controlled movements of tai chi produce amazing balance, strength, flexibility, and numerous anti-aging benefits. Two recent studies demonstrated the anti-aging benefits of tai chi.

In the first study, several anti-aging tests were done on 10 men (average age, 70 years) who had practiced tai chi 5 days a week for 11 years. The same tests were done on another group of 10 men of the same age who had not practiced tai chi. The men who practiced tai chi had 34 percent greater lung capacity (peak VO_2) than those who had not practiced tai chi. They also had better microcirculation in their extremities, which was presumed to be a result of greater nitric oxide release. It should be noted that nitric oxide is also a brain stimulant and a probable source of the balanced mental outlook produced by tai chi.

The second study measured bone mineral density (BMD) among 17 women ages 50 to 59 who had practiced tai chi daily for over 4 years. They were compared with 17 women of the same age who did not practice tai chi. BMD in weight-bearing bones among the tai chi group was 10 to 15 percent higher than in the non–tai chi group. Moreover, in follow-up studies 12 months later, the tai chi women experienced far less bone loss than their nonexercising counterparts.

Qi gong is a therapeutic Chinese practice that has been used for thousands of years to balance and restore body energy or *qi*. It seeks to harmonize mind, body, and spirit using exercises for the breath, mind, and voice. Although qi is a physical entity that practitioners of acupuncture can manipulate effectively, the concept is a little strange to Westerners. Can you really change the flow of energy in your body?

Researchers from the American College of Traditional Chinese Medicine in San Francisco, California, measured electrodermal conductance (Ryodoraku responses) among 29 subjects attending a 2-day workshop on qi gong. Electrical conductivity was measured in 24 acupuncture points on the wrists and feet of participants. Energy levels were less in the afternoon than in the morning and lower on the first day than the second. By the end of the second day, energy levels were actually higher in the afternoon and there was a better overall balance of energy (qi) between the various acupuncture points. Apparently, the training the attendees received was effective in an amazingly short time.

Another study on the effectiveness of qi gong to improve biopsychosocial health was done with a group of 50 geriatric patients in various stages of subacute chronic illness. Half of the participants took a 12-week course in qi gong while the other half attended their regular rehabilitation sessions. A questionnaire and informal biofeedback were used to evaluate the improvement in physical and psychological health, social relationship, and overall health. The qi gong group expressed improvement in all the biopsychosocial measures, whereas there was no improvement among those who continued the regular remedial treatment.

Yoga is a practice of meditative and physical exercises based on 2,000-year-old teachings in India. We briefly discussed yoga in chapter 3 as a meditative exercise. Here we explain the anti-aging effects of yoga exercises. In general, the anti-aging benefits enjoyed by yoga practitioners include improved respiratory capacity, lower blood pressure and heart rate, and lower cholesterol.

Yoga also improves nerve conduction in type 2 diabetics. Twenty diabetics ages 30 to 60 performed yoga exercises 30 to 40 minutes each morning for 40 days. The test subjects continued to take their medications and followed a low-glycemic diet. Another group of diabetics were also kept on medication and the prescribed diet. However, this group used light physical exercises such as walking instead of yoga. At the end of 40 days, the velocity of nerve conduction in the yoga group had increased significantly while the nerve conduction in the control group had deteriorated—a normal course of events in diabetics.

Additionally, yoga seems to increase handgrip strength even among those suffering from rheumatoid arthritis (RA). Handgrip strength was measured in 37 normal adults, 86 children, and 20 RA patients who were enrolled in yoga classes. Handgrip strength was measured at the beginning of the classes, which varied in duration (30 days for adults, 10 days for children, and 20 days for RA patients). Handgrip strength in a group of people with similar makeup who did not take the yoga classes (controls) was assessed for comparison. All of those who attended the yoga classes increased handgrip strength, with women both normal and with RA showing the greatest gains. The control group did not improve handgrip strength.

Yoga exercises are effective physical training for improving reaction time, motor skills, dexterity, muscle power, respiratory endurance, and visual perception and for reducing anxiety and aggression. Yoga is very effective for children and may help those who are struggling with behavioral problems. This was demonstrated with a group of girls raised in a community home.

The girls trained in yoga developed better muscle power, dexterity, positive attitude, and athletic skill than another group of girls in the same home who just did regular physical activities. These skills were also more developed among the yoga girls as compared with girls attending regular school and participating in a physical education program.

The Anti-Aging Exercise Prescription

The anti-aging exercise prescription involves three basic parts:

1. Stretching—improves flexibility and balance, reduces injury, relieves pain
2. Aerobic exercise—including warm-up, increases heart rate and lung capacity, begins releasing anti-aging hormones and neurotransmitters
3. Anaerobic exercise—builds strength and releases key anti-aging hormones: insulin, glucagon, human growth hormone (HGH), insulin-like growth factor 1 (IGF-1), and testosterone (also affected by diet as discussed in chapter 4)

The new government health guidelines recommend an hour of exercise a day—a goal that does not seem achievable to most people. However, ordinary tasks can make a significant contribution to the daily total. For example, you can do simple exercises while sitting at your desk.

Anti-aging exercises promote quality over quantity. We build strength by engaging small-muscle groups that are not normally accessed. We also use the large-muscle groups of the body for movement but with the emphasis on taking stress from joints. These exercises are based on the techniques of Joseph Pilates, who trained dancers, actors, and athletes in his New York studio. They emphasize building strength in the trunk muscles of the body, lower abdominals, obliques, and under the shoulder blades. Movement of muscle groups in the rest of the body begins first by engaging the core muscles (transverse abdominus) of the pelvis by drawing your navel to your spine.

Pilates stresses a neutral spine position that takes stress from the pelvis and back. To find neutral spine, lie on your back and tilt your pelvis first up and then down as much as you can. Find a relaxed middle position that allows you to slide a finger between your spine and the floor. Maintain this neutral spine position in standing, walking, and sitting.

Pilates also emphasizes keeping the shoulders relaxed. Upper body exercises are always generated by first sliding the shoulder blades down the back. Avoid squeezing shoulder blades together or letting shoulders hunch upward. This simple rule prevents neck, shoulder, and upper back tension and should be practiced throughout the day.

Floor mat exercises in Pilates and yoga are very similar. Pilates differs in that it makes use of a reformer for resistance training. This device uses a system of springs and pulleys attached to a base with a movable platform that provides varying degrees of resistance for working muscle groups without stressing any part of the body. We will discuss more about use of the Pilates reformer later. Now let's get started!

Basic Rules of Anti-Aging Exercise

As you have now seen, the new emphasis in anti-aging exercise is on building core stability and strength, then working the rest of the body from this center. Check out these basic rules of Pilates. You'll quickly see why they confer amazing anti-aging benefits.

- Always start your exercise session with stretching and a warm-up.
- Take your time. The slower you do these exercises, the better.
- Move in rhythm with your breathing.
- Exert muscle movement as you exhale. Relax as you inhale.
- As you begin each movement, first draw your navel to your spine.
- Keep checking your posture. The Pilates posture emphasizes standing tall, yet relaxed and comfortable.
- Stay focused on what your body is doing even when you're not exercising. This is how you'll turn ordinary tasks into exercise.
- Build up abdominal strength slowly. Engage your lower transverse abdominal muscles (seat-belt muscles) and don't allow your "six-pack" (abdominal muscles) to bulge.
- Move your arms and shoulders by generating movement from the group of muscles over your shoulder blades (teres major and minor, supraspinatus, infraspinatus) and large back muscles (latissimus dorsi or "lats"). Avoid hunching your shoulders and squeezing your shoulder blades together (trapezius). Focus on keeping shoulders low and relaxed throughout the day.
- Keep repetitions low. Quality, not quantity, is what counts. Pilates typically uses 4 or 8 repetitions. If you find you're "powering" through your exercises—stop! (See the Massachusetts YMCA study below.)
- Perform the exercises regularly—ideally every other day.
- Above all, persevere.
- We are using the Pilates as our anti-aging fitness model. You should incorporate these exercises into whatever other exercise you choose. Use Pilates rules in the workplace and in everything else you do.

Speed Isn't the Answer!

Sports medicine doctors in Massachusetts enrolled 65 men and 82 women with an average age of 53 years in a 13-week training program at the local YMCA. None of the study enrollees had previously lifted weights. All participants trained on a 13-circuit Nautilus doing either regular speed lifts of 8 to 10 reps at 7 seconds each (2 seconds lifting, 1 second pause, 4 seconds lowering), or superslow at 4 to 6 reps at 14 seconds each (10 seconds lifting, 4 seconds lowering). Amazingly, the superslow reps produced a 50 percent greater increase in muscle strength in both men and women than regular-speed reps. The researchers advised physicians to tell middle-age and older adults to slow down when they exercise.

This study demonstrates the wisdom of methods used by Joseph Pilates and ancient movement exercises such as yoga, tai chi, and qi gong for anti-aging benefits. There are many interpretations of the work that Joseph Pilates did. We list several books and videotapes on Pilates, yoga, tai chi, and qi gong in the resources section.

Learning these techniques is very helpful not only because they help produce a trim, lithe body with impressive muscle definition but also because they can turn ordinary activities into meaningful exercise. They will also help you get more out of your gym workout as we'll show you later in this chapter.

These exercises involve relearning how to move. Move very slowly as you become accustomed to accessing forgotten muscles. As the movements become more automatic, you can pick up speed.

Breathing Exercises

Taking time to check your breathing will help prevent fatigue, reduce irritation, and keep you focused. If possible, it helps to close your eyes while you take three or four slow deep breaths.

- Practice thoracic breathing. This means pulling air deeply into the back of your lungs, taking care to not let your ribs flare in front.
- Inhale through your nose as you relax. Yoga teaches you how to inhale through the nostril on one side, then switch to the other, in order to better access your autonomic nervous system.
- Exhale slowly through your mouth as you expel most of the volume of air in your lungs.
- Take a breathing break several times a day or whenever stressed.

Benefits of Breathing Exercise

Exercise (15 minutes)	⇨ Stimulates lympatic and blood flow ⇨ Stretches leg joints and muscles ⇨ Helps balance sympathetic and parasympathetic nervous systems
Breathing (5 minutes)	⇨ Improves flow of blood to stem of brain and major organs ⇨ Balances acid and base levels of blood

The benefits of deep breathing can be felt even without exercise. However, the benefits increase when correct breathing is incorporated into exercise.

Warm-Up Exercises

Simple daily stretching exercises can keep you loose and flexible. Your daily exercise routine should improve the range of motion in your major joints, giving you a feeling of confidence, helping you to gain more pleasure in exercising, and reducing the possibility of injury.

David Thomas, M.D., of Mt. Sinai School of Medicine, says: "Range of motion decreases if you don't use your major joints. With disuse, muscles and tendons contract and make the joints feel stiff. As a result, they can't easily move through their full range of motion. The longer a joint remains fixed, the harder it is to reverse the effect."

Stretching is important in nervous system regulation. It normalizes neurotransmitter function through the motion generated by inner ear stimulation. That's why we suggest you close your eyes if at all possible when doing exercises for stretching and balance. It enhances the effect of stretching by activating nerve and hormone centers. *Focus on Healthy Healing,* the newsletter of Mt. Sinai Medical School, advises: "Start slowly, performing each exercise a few times only and then increase to 8 or 10 reps. When stretching, go to the point where you feel a noticeable stretching sensation, but don't force it. Back it off if you feel pain."

Stretching "primes" your body for exercise. It is also a good practice to use throughout the day for improving balance between activating reactions (sympathetic) and calming ones (parasympathetic).

Benefits of Stretching Exercise

	Benefits	**Type of Exercise**
Sympathetic Tone Parasympathetic	⇨ Flexibility ⇨ Improved organ perfusion ⇨ Improved autonomic function	⇨ Yoga ⇨ Stretching ⇨ Pilates mat exercises

Flexibility and Stretching Exercises

Neck

There are four simple neck flexibility exercises you can do in the workplace or at home. These help reduce tension on your shoulders and improve circulation to your brain.

- Alternate stretching your neck by looking up to the ceiling, then tuck your chin into your chest. Concentrate on making your neck as long as possible. Computer users may find massaging the tendons that run along the back of the neck (cervical) vertebra extremely helpful. Use your right fingers to slide over the left cervical tendon while pressing on it. Use your left fingers for the right side. You can apply pressure until you feel the tendon "pop" as it moves slightly under the pressure. You can press along several locations—first at the base of your skull, then farther down toward your neck. Find which position seems to relieve neck tension the best.
- Tilt your right ear toward your right shoulder, then repeat on the left side. Be extremely careful to not scrunch your shoulders. Try to drop your shoulder down as you tilt your head toward it. Watch that you don't lift the opposite shoulder.
- Rotate your head slowly to the left, then to the right. You will feel a good stretch in your neck muscles as you do this. Always avoid the tendency to lift your shoulders.
- Stand comfortably with your arms outstretched at shoulder height. Rotate your head slowly clockwise, letting your head fall as far to the front, back, and sides as you can without having your shoulders or back tense up. Repeat 8 times. Reverse direction to counterclockwise and repeat the exercise. Closing your eyes while you do this adds difficulty.

Shoulders

We have been stressing throughout this chapter the importance of keeping your shoulders loose. Tense shoulders increase tension throughout your body and can cause headaches, some vision problems, and mental and physical fatigue.

- Place the back of your hand, thumb up, against your back at waist height. Slowly slide your hand along your spine toward your upper back. Get your hand as close to your shoulders as possible without tensing your shoulders or back. Repeat with the other hand. This exercise can be repeated throughout the day.
- Using flexible rubber tubing or a band, you can apply isometric exercises to strengthen the rotator cuff on the inside of your shoulders. Attach one end of the rubber tubing to a closed-door knob. Grab the band with one fist, keeping your upper arm pressed against your side. Your elbow should be bent at 90 degrees, with your forearm extending 90 degrees in front of your body. Slowly stretch the band across the front of your waist as you flatten your fist against your body, keeping your upper arm glued to your side. Be sure and keep your wrists straight. This will be a lever action across the front of your body that only involves your forearm and hand. Repeat on the other side. Do this 8 times. As you gain strength and flexibility, you can increase tension on the band by grasping it closer to the door handle.
- With both elbows at your waist in the same 90-degree position as above, grab the rubber band between your fists and stretch it across the front of your body by turning your wrists at right angles to your body. Keep your upper arms firmly glued to your sides. This is also a lever action, extending just your forearms and hands away from your body. Do 8 repetitions.

Lower Back

Most exercise books have excellent stretching exercises for your lower back. We offer these because they are some of the best for office workers.

- Lie down on the carpet or exercise mat on your back. Draw your knees to your chest as closely as you can and still feel loose. Grasp your wrists around your shins and roll from side to side to loosen up your lower back. Just roll slowly from side to side for a few seconds without rolling over onto your side. Closing your eyes as you roll will enhance the relaxation and stretching benefits. Do this and the following lower back exercises every morning to wake up and in the evening to let go of your day.

- While still on your back, put the soles of your feet together, reach between your bent knees, and hold your feet with your hands. Your knees will be spread wide to relax your hips. Roll from side to side, tightening your core muscles to control the movement and keep from rolling over. Do this 8 times, closing your eyes if possible.
- Next, bring your legs back together folded close to your chest and grasp your wrists around your shins. Tuck your head, round your spine, and begin rolling your spine along the mat while staying in a tight roll. Do easy rolls forward and backward to relax your spine. Be sure to keep your back rounded so that you protect your spine. Begin with little momentum rolls, gradually increasing them to bring your entire back in contact with the mat. These three exercises warm up your spine and should be done before you attempt any other exercise.
- Sit up tall and extend your legs out straight in front of you with your feet flexed. Your feet should be in a straight line with your hips. Reach forward as far as you can, touching your toes if possible. Hold the stretch as you count to 8. This exercise can also be done with a rubber band or towel. The idea is to get a good stretch for the muscles along the back of your leg.
- In the same sitting position, extend your legs wide apart in a straddle position in front of you. Now touch your left toes, or as far down your leg as possible, reaching across your body with your right hand. Hold the stretch for 8. Now you will feel the muscles in your side (obliques) getting stretched as well. Be sure and keep your shoulders relaxed and core tight. Repeat on the other side.
- Now curl up with your legs folded under you and arms extended along the floor in front of you. Drop your head as low to the floor as possible. Just hang out there for 8 seconds feeling the stretch along your entire curled back and legs. Roll over to your side and get up.

Hips

Loss of flexibility happens in any joint that isn't worked out regularly. Loss of flexion in hips is especially dangerous because it leads to loss of balance and the possibility of falling, twisting, spraining, or breaking a leg, ankle, or foot. Falls are a major cause of hip fracture in those over age 75, and they can often be prevented by hip stretches done throughout life.

- While standing, grab the back of a chair or counter top. Slowly draw one leg toward your chest, bending your knee until it reaches a 90-degree angle. Keep the foot on the supporting leg tracking straight ahead, the foot on the lifting leg flexed. Pull your navel to your spine and you do so and breathe. Repeat 4 to 8 times and then go to the other side. As you become more accomplished at this, close your eyes while doing the exercise. You can also keep your foot lower and let go of the chair or counter. This exercise improves balance. See Chapter 3, the test you did for static balance.
- In the same position, slowly lift your leg back behind you, tightening your gluts and keeping your knee as straight as possible, as you do so. Keep your foot flexed. Repeat 4 to 8 times and then go to the other side.
- Keeping this same starting position, now lift your straight leg out to the side. Again, keep your leg straight and foot flexed. Move it slowly up and down 4 to 8 times. Repeat on the other side. Keep your body tall and straight as you do these exercises. Engage your core and avoid tensing your shoulders or leaning to one side.

Legs

Walking and other forms of exercise discussed below improve circulation of blood and lymph. So will taking walking breaks in the office. However, you can exercise your legs while sitting, even in cramped airline spaces.

- While sitting and with your knees at a 90-degree angle, lift the front of your feet so that your feet are resting on their heels. Lift and drop the front of your feet so that the muscles on the front of your leg are worked. Do this 4 to 8 times. Next, rotate your feet outward, Charlie Chaplin style, and do the same series of foot lifts. Notice how different muscles in the front of your leg are worked. Now turn your toes so that they are touching (kissing) and you're slightly knock-kneed. Repeat the foot lifts. You can get a nice rhythm going with these foot lifts if you first lift one, then the other, in a modified treading motion. Add the treading motion to all three foot positions.

- Still sitting, stretch your legs out in front of you (you may not be able to do this on the airplane!). Repeat the foot lifts and drops, first with your feet pointing straight ahead, then Charlie Chaplin style, followed by toes kissing. The amazing thing is that just by turning your feet, you access forgotten little muscles that will strengthen your ankles, feet, and legs.
- When you are someplace where you have a wider range of motion, try these same foot lifts with your legs raised higher. Try them first with your legs straight ahead, then with your legs wide in a straddle.
- Finish these exercises with a good stretch for the back of your legs by lifting your legs as high as you can, being careful to tighten your core and breathe. You can use a rubber exercise band for these exercises. Standing tall with your legs hip-width apart, slowly hinge forward from the hips and touch your toes, or as low as you can reach. Try keeping your back as straight as possible, like dancers do. Hold your bend for 8 seconds to give the back of your legs a good stretch.

Advantages of Exercising at Home

Americans are urged to take up a regular exercise program to fight the growing obesity problem. But should you exercise at home or do you need to go to a gym?

Researchers at the University of Florida in Gainesville enrolled 49 obese women in a yearlong behavioral weight-loss program. All participants engaged in moderate-intensity walking for 30 minutes a day, 5 days per week. Half of the women participated in three supervised group exercise sessions per week for 6 months, then two times per week for the remaining 6 months of the study. The second half of the group did their prescribed exercise at home.

At the end of 6 months, all of the women displayed significant improvement in exercise participation, fitness, eating patterns, and weight loss. At 12 months, the home-based group showed superior adherence to an exercise schedule, and at 15 months they also demonstrated much greater weight loss than the group exercisers. Exercising at home offers many advantages, and you can enhance the anti-aging benefits by getting as much exercise at work as possible.

Exercises for the Workplace

Many of us spend most of the workday sitting, so we need to include sitting exercises as part of our anti-aging program. The following exercises will help make you much more productive at work and reduce fatigue and stress:

- Sit tall with a neutral spine (small curve in your middle back, hips level).
- Comfortably space your legs at a 90-degree angle and in alignment with your hips.
- Point your feet straight ahead so that they are aligned with your knees.
- Button your navel to your spine, reducing pressure on your back.
- Place a 4-inch foam ball between your knees to help maintain position without having to think about it. Squeeze the ball with your inner thigh muscles from time to time to strengthen them and improve circulation.
- Keep your shoulders low and relaxed with a wide collarbone. Slide your shoulder blades down from time to time, exhaling as you do so. Be sure not to pinch your shoulder blades together. This exercise is extremely important for avoiding carpal tunnel syndrome and neck strain.
- Keep your computer keyboard at elbow level so that it is comfortable for your arms and wrists. This is also important for reducing stress to the elbows and wrists.
- Keep a workout band in your desk to use for stretching, strengthening, and improving circulation
- Get up from your chair frequently and take a walk around the office. Take the stairs, if possible.

Exercising in short bouts throughout the day can be just as effective as doing it all at one time. British researchers wanted to see if a group of young female sedentary office workers could benefit from taking the stairs instead of the elevator. Twenty-two women were divided into two groups. One group started climbing stairs at work and the other group stayed at their desks. The stair-climbers started with just one ascent of 199 steps the first few days, then worked their way up to six ascents by the end of the 7-week trial. Oxygen uptake and heart rate were monitored continuously during ascent, and blood lactate was measured immediately after each ascent. Blood samples were taken from both groups and analyzed for serum lipids. There were few changes among the desk-sitting group, whereas the stair-climbers displayed a rise in healthy HDL cholesterol and an improved ratio between HDL and unhealthy LDL cholesterol. Oxygen uptake, heart rate, and blood lactate were all reduced among the stair-climbing group. So, instead of heading for the coffee-break room, grab some water and head for the stairs. Be sure to maximize your muscle work as you climb. Breathe in as you step up and breathe out as you shift your weight upward, using your breath to help engage glut and thigh muscles.

We're emphasizing the newest thinking in anti-aging exercise—that working smart means moving your body from a position of strength, being careful to maintain a strong core. That's where the stability aspect of the plan comes in. We also emphasize consistency and bringing your exercise techniques into as many of your daily activities as possible.

Many people who work in cities have already discovered the importance of walking during lunch hour. Nevertheless, did you know there's a big difference between power walking and anti-aging walking?

Anti-Aging Walking

Anti-aging walking develops strength, stability, and mind fitness. Problems with hips, knees, and feet are extremely common as we age. Anti-aging walking protects against these problems because it strengthens large- and small-muscle groups that take the load from the knees. By keeping your seat-belt muscles engaged and a neutral spine, you will strengthen your back. Proper tracking with your feet straight ahead helps strengthen your arches and reduce foot problems. And, you will be so busy concentrating on how you're moving that you won't have time to ruminate over work problems.

Walking is one of the best anti-aging exercises. You are probably aware of the cardiovascular benefits of walking, but you may not know that walking affects levels of several hormones, burns fat, and reduces food intake because your body switches to utilizing stored body fat for fuel instead of glucose. A long-term walking program leads to fat loss without dieting. Regular walking reduces insulin requirements, with approximately a 36 percent decrease in the ratio of insulin to glucose.

Before eating breakfast, get in 20 minutes of walking. This helps reset your metabolic rate, allowing you to burn off excess calories and fats consumed the previous day. Walking has a powerful effect on hormones, enhancing growth hormone levels, reducing cortisol levels, and speeding up the rate of nutrient delivery to your cells.

On the Internet, check out America on the Move (www. americaonthemove.org), the latest campaign to get Americans moving. Buy a step counter and try to add an additional 2,000 steps, or about 1 mile, to your daily routine.

Plan 20 minutes in the middle of your workday for a walk, and don't walk more than 40 minutes. This may be in addition to or in place of your morning or evening walk. Many cities have beautiful urban parks that are great for walking. Get some coworkers to join you and become part of the latest fitness trend.

Begin slowly so that you can concentrate on maximizing muscle work and breathing. As you become more proficient, you will be able to walk faster. Remember, quality is what you're after, not quantity or speed.

Start with a pair of good supportive shoes that have no heels. Most brands of sport shoes have designs for walking. Wear sport socks to cushion your feet and wick away moisture. Before you leave the office, stretch the muscles in the back of your legs and do a few knee bends to warm up your quads. Drink 8 ounces of water before heading out. If the weather is warm, take a bottle of water with you.

Walking on a flat street works all the muscle groups in your lower body from the navel down. It keeps the shoulders and lower arms relaxed while working the upper arms.

For the upper body, keep your shoulders low and neck long. Swing your arms comfortably at your side, elbows slightly bent, alternating with elbows bent at 90 degrees and hands slightly in front of your abdomen. Keep a neutral spine and eyes ahead. Avoid checking out the display windows in stores you pass! Breathe deeply!

For the lower body, keep seat-belt muscles engaged and concentrate on using your quads, internal thigh muscles, gluts, and hamstrings. Alternately contract and relax these muscles as you walk. Watch your foot tracking. Balance on the three points of your feet: the heels and outer and inner balls. Be sure your feet are pointing straight ahead. A natural swing of your waist and hips occurs as you walk. Pretty soon you'll need a smaller belt!

Walking on hills is a series of alternating flexing and stretching exercises. If you have hills near work or home, you are very fortunate. As you walk uphill, stretch your legs as you push off behind your body. Feel the pull on your heels, hamstrings (back of your thighs), calf muscles, and hips. As you step uphill, concentrate on flexing your quads (front of thighs), calves, gluts (buttocks), and feet. Extend your legs behind you as you push uphill with your back foot in order to get the maximum stretch. You will also feel the muscles in the front of your shins engaging as you lift your feet. Your hips will get a good stretch as you walk uphill. Keep your seat-belt muscles engaged and move your arms with a 90-degree bend in your elbows. Resist the temptation to shrug your shoulders. Keep eyes ahead and focus on how you are engaging your muscles.

As you walk downhill, take as much pressure off your knees as possible by increasing the bend of your knees and tightening your gluts. Downhill walking emphasizes your thigh muscles (quads). You can utilize your gluts and to a lesser degree your calf muscles to stabilize your body, particularly on steep hills. Go slowly as if you have a great load on your back. Watch foot tracking and shoulders. You will naturally lean slightly back, but keep seat-belt muscles engaged to eliminate strain on your spine.

Inhale deeply through your nose, pulling air into your lungs toward your spine. Avoid letting your rib cage stick out in front, as this automatically causes you to tense your shoulders. Draw in air toward your core, energizing your center of strength. Exhale slowly through slightly pursed lips. Develop your own natural rhythm of inhaling and exhaling every few steps.

Most people walk for cardio conditioning and to burn calories. Anti-aging walking has both of these benefits. You will be working larger calorie-guzzling muscles while improving the shape of your body. And as these muscles work, they consume more energy and blood, improving cardiovascular fitness. You don't have to huff and puff to gain these benefits. However, as you become more proficient in anti-aging walking skills, you can pick up the pace. If you are losing weight as you progress in your walking, you will have to step up the pace anyway. Packing fewer pounds burns less energy. If you enjoy speed walking, just make sure you don't hunch your shoulders as you step along, and avoid hyperextending your knees. Speed walking utilizes more lateral work as your hips rotate with the stiff-legged gait. It is an excellent way to develop a trim midsection and tight gluts. Speed walking is best done in a park or someplace where you won't be interrupted by traffic.

How you walk is extremely important in getting the maximum anti-aging benefits. Epidemiologists at the Michigan Department of Community Health reported that less then 40 percent of walkers complied with the most liberal standards for physical activity. To get the full anti-aging benefits of walking, you should either walk briskly and more frequently using the techniques we have given you here or engage in a complementary physical activity such as weight training.

Following your walk with a few simple weight-bearing exercises when you return to work can add additional benefits. They may be isometric exercises using an exercise rubber band. And best of all, you don't need a lot of expensive equipment to achieve startling results. In fact, you may do more harm than good if you use equipment improperly. What's more, you can sabotage your anti-aging gains by doing the wrong exercises for your genes.

Why Overtraining Ages You

Exercise only until you feel stress on your joints and regardless of whether you are stretching or lifting weights. Stop if your muscles begin to severely quiver. It's normal for muscles that haven't been exercised in a while to be weak, but be extremely careful not to overdo it. You may be surprised how little strength you have in your smaller stabilizing muscles.

Heavy exercise for more than 40 minutes at a time or exercise that burns more than 2,000 calories a week actually sabotages your anti-aging program by increasing oxidative stress and raising cortisol levels. First, you'll be increasing free radical generation as mitochondria pump out energy to sustain the work you're doing. Second, cortisol levels will surge as you push your body into fight-or-flight mode. In fact, exercising strenuously for more than 45 minutes causes cortisol levels to rise so high that levels of other hormones including testosterone and growth hormone drop, and other hormone functions are impaired.

An increase in cortisol causes an increase in blood glucose, resulting in an increase in insulin levels. Testosterone production declines as testosterone precursors shift to making more cortisol.

Antioxidants and other supplements (chapter 6) become a necessity for those involved in intense training. You'll need recovery time to reduce cortisol levels and attention to the anti-aging meals plans (chapter 4) to keep insulin under control and to help offset the deleterious effects if you overtrain. Finally, you should monitor your hormone levels with the saliva test kit we suggest in appendix A. Based on the tests suggested in appendix A, you may need to balance hormones through the methods we discuss in chapter 7.

Benefits of Aerobic Exercise

	Benefits	**Type of Exercise**
Aerobic (cardiovascular)	Heart and vascular system Fat burning	⇨ Biking ⇨ Walking ⇨ Running ⇨ Jogging

Aerobic Exercise

Aerobic exercise increases breathing, circulation, and heart rate. It activates hormones that burn fat and improve mental outlook. Aerobic exercise shifts metabolism away from storing fat into burning it. At the beginning of exercise, you're priming your muscles as well as your cardiovascular and respiratory systems for increased activity. A sequence of events occurs during aerobic exercise.

During the first 20 minutes of exercise, your body shifts from burning glucose to burning stored glycogen as the primary fuel, which is better suited to providing energy for working muscles. Insulin is not required for mobilizing glycogen, so levels of the hormone drop. At the same time, your body begins releasing growth hormone (HGH), which repairs muscle and increases its mass while bumping up fat burning.

During the next 40 minutes, exercise progresses as you move into anaerobic (weight-bearing) exercise. Glycogen stores become depleted and fat becomes your primary fuel, with a steady release of glucose from both of these fuels. At the end of 45 minutes, HGH levels begin to drop off. The ideal time to begin resistance work is before HGH levels decline. This will be following your 20-minute aerobic (cardio) exercise.

The events that take place during aerobic exercise—namely a decrease in insulin levels, an increase in HGH and fat burning—prepare your body for maximum benefits from your resistance workout. In addition, aerobic exercise improves cardiovascular and respiratory function, thereby conferring tremendous anti-aging benefits. Aerobic exercise also develops stamina and improves balance and coordination.

Cycling is enjoyed by a growing number of enthusiasts. A research team at the University of Utah wanted to know if mountain biking or road biking conferred more anti-aging benefits and how these sports compared to other forms of exercise. Muscle strength and power, aerobic fitness, bone mineral density, and sex hormone data were collected

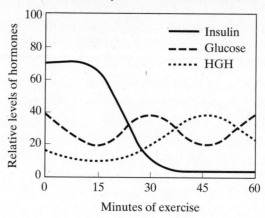

Hormonal Response to Aerobic Exercise

Minutes of exercise

on 30 competitive cyclists, ages 20 to 40, half of them mountain cyclists and the other half road warriors.

The data gathered from the cyclists were compared with those obtained from 15 recreationally active men of the same age. The only measurement that was significantly different among the three groups was bone mineral density, which was much greater among mountain cyclists. It would seem that all those jolts and bumps imposed by this sport stimulate the formation of dense bones.

Significant benefits from other less strenuous forms of aerobic fitness have also been shown. Two studies—one done at Loma Linda University in Loma Linda, California, and the other at the University of Kuopio in Kuopio, Finland—found that light to moderate exercise protected men from cardiovascular disease. The Loma Linda group analyzed data from 44,452 male health professionals. They found that moderate participation in aerobic and anaerobic exercise significantly reduced incidence of cardiac events. Men who ran for an hour or more per week had a 42 percent risk reduction. Those who trained with weights 30 minutes or more per week had a 23 percent reduction, and those who rowed for an hour or walked a half hour per day had an 18 percent reduction in risk.

The Finnish researchers studied the benefits of leisure-time physical activity (golf, gardening) in preventing cardiovascular disease and metabolic syndrome (insulin insensitivity, diabetes). Among 612 middle-age men, those who engaged in at least 3 hours per week of activity were half as likely as sedentary men to develop metabolic syndrome.

Vigorous leisure-time activity had even greater benefits. Men who ranked in the upper third of oxygen intake (VO_2 max), had a 75 percent lower risk than sedentary men of developing metabolic syndrome.

Other amazing benefits seen among both men and women engaging in aerobic fitness include lowered risk of upper respiratory infection and reduced incapacity from carpal tunnel syndrome. Water aerobics increased cardiorespiratory fitness and muscular strength as well as decreased body fat and total cholesterol in older adult women. Similarly, yard work that involves lifting and carrying loads appears to build denser bones than jogging, swimming, cycling, aerobics, walking, dancing, and calisthenics. Only weight training had the same positive benefits as yard work.

Scientists at Auburn University in Alabama wanted to know if 8 weeks of aerobic dance using weights would increase VO_2 max and body composition among 28 coeds. Half the group danced with weights and the other half did the same exercises but did not use weights. While handheld weights did not cause additional pain and stiffness, they also did not increase the workload sufficiently to boost VO_2 max or improve body composition over what was seen in those not using weights. Other researchers have reported mixed benefits from using handheld weights. It appears you are better off choosing a separate activity for anaerobic benefits.

Anaerobic Exercise

Anaerobic exercise continues the release of growth hormone when it follows aerobic exercise. The rise in HGH is accompanied by increasing testosterone levels. Resistance exercise develops muscles, improves body composition, and increases bone density and overall body strength. Again, we see a sequence of events in hormone release during anaerobic exercise.

Benefits of Resistive Exercise

	Benefits	Type of Exercise
Resistive (anaerobic)	Muscle toning Muscle building	⇨ Weight ⇨ Pilates ⇨ Calisthenics

For the first 30 minutes, HGH and testosterone levels increase, peaking at 30 minutes. Anaerobic exercise increases levels of these hormones more than aerobic exercise. The drop in insulin that began during aerobic conditioning continues. Doing more than 30 to 40 minutes of heavy exercise will not boost hormone levels higher.

After 30 minutes of anaerobic exercise, levels of testosterone and HGH begin declining, although the effects of increased HGH and testosterone on the body continue. It is during this period that muscle tone and mass improve, and tendon and ligament strength is developed. Insulin levels continue to remain low.

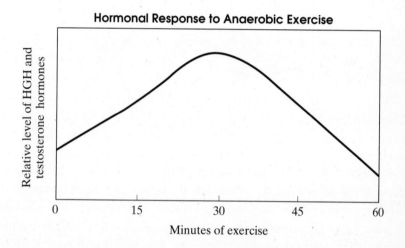

Hormonal Response to Anaerobic Exercise

It is apparent that the most ideal exercise plan includes

- 20 to 30 minutes of aerobic exercise followed by 30 to 40 minutes of resistance exercise
- Stretching and warm-up before exercise and cooldown and release afterward
- Breathing correctly through the exercises

The following diagram gives an integrated picture of what's happening during aerobic and anaerobic exercise and how the two kinds of exercise provide overall anti-aging benefits. The drop in blood glucose and insulin is accompanied by an increase in HGH and testosterone. Women benefit from increases in these hormones just as men do. Testosterone is present in both genders and has the same beneficial effect of increasing bone density and muscle strength. In women, these effects are moderated by estrogen and progesterone, so resistance training doesn't produce bulging muscles.

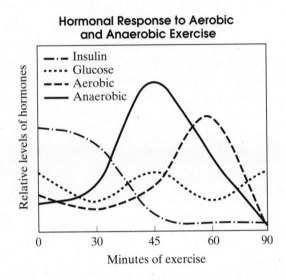

Hormonal Response to Aerobic and Anaerobic Exercise

A team of scientists and trainers at the University of Maryland in College Park compared the effects of strength training between young and older people. The study included 8 men and 6 women ages 20 to 30 and 9 men and 10 women ages 65 to 75 in a 6-month strength-training program that worked all major muscle groups. Muscle size of thighs and quadriceps increased significantly in all participants regardless of gender or age. This study demonstrates that strength training can be just as effective for older people as younger ones.

Moreover, resistance training is very effective in improving body shape, particularly in older women. Scientists at the University of Alabama in Birmingham recruited 12 women and 14 men ages 61 to 77 in a 6-month resistance-training program. By the end of the training period, the women had gained between 22 and 38 percent muscle strength and lost a substantial amount of abdominal fat, particularly subcutaneous belly fat. The men also gained between 21 and 36 percent muscle strength and lost body fat. However, subcutaneous abdominal fat was not reduced in the men. Despite gender differences in body sculpting between women and men, gains in strength and fat loss are positively associated with anti-aging benefits.

It has been recognized for many years that aerobic exercise

improves insulin response and glucose tolerance, which are both important factors in preventing insulin resistance and non-insulin-dependent diabetes mellitus. A research team from the University of Texas at Austin reviewed recent studies to determine what specific effects anaerobic exercise could offer for preventing insulin resistance. They found that anaerobic exercise actually changes the composition and activity of muscle fibers, increasing uptake of glucose into muscles and enzyme activity that converts glucose into energy. Specifically, they found that the activities of two types of fast-twitch muscle fibers are modified by anaerobic exercise. Fast-twitch muscle fibers are those that can produce energy from glucose quickly but tire easily. Type IIa muscle fibers are more insulin sensitive than type IIb fibers, meaning that they require less insulin to process glucose efficiently. Anaerobic exercise increases their activity and number, resulting in improved glucose tolerance and lowered fasting insulin levels.

More recently, Australian scientists studied the effect of anaerobic exercise on older overweight individuals with type 2 diabetes. Thirty-six men and women between the ages of 60 and 80 were enrolled in a 6-month program that included weight loss and either resistance training or mild exercise (control group). Both groups lost weight and fat mass. However, the resistance group gained lean body mass while the control group lost muscle mass. Since diabetes causes loss of muscle, a resistance training program is essential to improving this condition.

Exercise by itself has not been found to substantially lower cholesterol levels unless the exercise is very intense. And, as we grow older, intense exercise may sabotage anti-aging goals. However, a new study has found that while levels of cholesterol may not be reduced by exercise alone, exercise may make cholesterol less dangerous. Doctors at Duke University and East Carolina University enrolled 85 men and women in an 8-month exercise program that involved moderate to light exercise. The subjects were told to eat as much as they needed to maintain current weight. Two-thirds of the subjects either jogged or walked the equivalent of 12 miles per week while the remaining third jogged the equivalent of 20 miles per week. The 12-mile exercise groups had significant changes in cholesterol particle size, increasing the number of large and less dangerous particles. These larger, fluffy particles are less likely to clog arteries than smaller, denser ones. The 20-mile group had even more pronounced positive changes. The results were determined by a new kind of blood test that differentiates between cholesterol-carrying protein particles. Although this test (nuclear magnetic resonance spectroscopy) is currently two to three times more expensive than standard blood tests and is done only in large medical centers, it may soon become more available and affordable. Such a definitive test would provide useful information for anti-aging. Be sure and check with your doctor for availability.

Both men and women lose bone mass as they get older. The effect is most pronounced among those who are sedentary. Could anaerobic exercise reverse bone loss and increase strength in older people? Doctors at the University of Florida, Gainesville, assigned 62 men and women ages 60 to 83 years to either of two exercise groups for 6 months of progressive resistance training. One group trained three times per week at 50 percent of the maximum reps they could do for 13 repetitions (low intensity). The other group trained three times per week at 80 percent of maximum reps for 8 repetitions (high intensity). At the end of 6 months, the gains in strength were about the same for both groups. However, only the high-intensity group gained bone mass and increased osteocalcin, a measure of bone mineral uptake.

At the Mayo Clinic in Rochester, Minnesota, 50 healthy women ages 58 to 75 were part of a bone density study on the effects of strengthening back muscles with resistive exercise. Half of the women performed resistive back exercises for 2 years and the other half didn't. At the end of 2 years, the exercising women substantially increased muscle strength in their backs. The nonexercising women did not increase back muscle strength and neither group increased bone density. Surprisingly, the exercising women had increased bone density 8 years later, even though they were no longer doing the back exercises, and back strength had dropped. Occurrence of compression fractures among both groups of women revealed that the nonexercise group had 2.7 times greater incidence of vertebral fracture. Amazingly, there were long-term benefits of resistive exercise on bone density, even years after discontinuance of exercise.

Scientists at Wake Forest University in Winston-Salem, North Carolina, conducted a 30-month study of 480 men and women age 65 or older with chronic knee pain. Researchers measured balance and strength of knee flexion and extension and ankle strength. Body mass index was also taken into account in determining degree of chronic knee pain. Subjects with the greatest knee and ankle strength experienced the least pain and loss of balance. Weight training has been established as an important part of therapy for improving balance and osteoarthritis in older adults. Maintenance of strong ankles, feet, and knees is an important part of anti-aging exercise.

American College of Sports Medicine Guidelines

The American College of Sports Medicine (ACSM) has published guidelines for anaerobic exercise. The guidelines emphasize quality, as we have done throughout this chapter.

- Exercise large muscle groups before concentrating on smaller ones.
- Multiple-joint exercises such as full arm or leg movements should be done before single joints such as elbows or shoulders.
- Higher-intensity exercises should be done before lower-intensity ones.
- For novices, weight loading should be appropriate to sustain a maximum of 8 to 12 repetitions, and training should take place 2 to 3 days a week.
- More advanced training should include a wider range of loads for 1 to 12 reps, eventually working up to heavier loads. Training should take place 4 to 5 days a week.
- ACSM established categories of weight lifting goals: weight lifting for muscle building, power training, and local muscle endurance training.

    Muscle building: The suggested guidelines are

    1. Increase load 2 to 10 percent when you can achieve 2 more than the desired number of reps. The desired number of reps is 6 to 12.
    2. Begin training 2 to 3 days per week and increase to 4 to 5 days per week.
    3. Take a 1- to 2-minute rest between sets.
    4. Use moderate-contraction velocity.

    Power training: The suggested guidelines are

    1. Use light loads, 30 to 60 percent of maximum repetitions.
    2. Use multiple reps to emphasize strength training.
    3. Take a 2- to 3-minute rest between sets.

4. Begin training 2 to 3 days per week and increase to 4 to 5 days per week.
5. Use fast-contraction velocity.

Local muscular endurance training: The suggested guidelines are

1. Use light to moderate loads, 40 to 60 percent of maximum repetitions.
2. Do at least 15 reps.
3. Take short rest periods—less than 90 seconds.

Resistance Training with Pilates

Athletic teams including professional football and basketball players and world-class golfers are turning to Pilates for training because it conditions forgotten small-muscle groups while larger muscles become increasingly toned and conditioned. Pilates never overtaxes your body, yet you will be surprised at what a good workout you get. The overall enhancement of a balanced body and one that is incredibly strong, agile, and flexible is very enviable. Accessing these smaller-muscle groups requires concentration, control, and precision that synchronize mind and body. Pilates has often been called the thinking exercise for this reason. Rather than powering through workouts, you will be using your mind to control muscle movement and you will be paying attention to how muscles are working.

Pilates is an incredible tool for rehabilitation from injuries, putting less stress on injured joints while building strength in the muscle groups that support them. Not surprisingly, it is a favorite among professional athletes, dancers, gymnasts, and skaters.

Pilates resistance training makes use of specialized equipment called a reformer, which consists of a platform with pulleys, spring weights, and a movable platform. The machine allows endless possibilities for working muscles and increasing workload by adjusting spring weights and direction of body motion so that different muscles are constantly being recruited. For example, just changing the position of hands and feet recruits a different set of muscles. Use of simple accessories in the mat and reformer exercises increases the anti-aging benefits. The moving platform on the reformer increases the benefit of resistance exercises as demonstrated by a recent study. A group of eight college men were studied for strength gains from doing curl-ups on a stable surface or using different positions on a movable surface such as the reformer platform.

Abdominal strength was increased by 21 percent and oblique muscle strength was increased by 5 percent when the men did their curl-ups on a stable surface. However, when doing curl-ups using three different moving positions, abdominal strength increased by 35 percent and oblique muscle strength increased by 10 percent. Moreover, the external oblique muscle gains were most pronounced using the movable surface.

PRESCRIPTION FOR ANTI-AGING EXERCISE IN THE GYM

Stretching	Aerobic Cardiovascular Training 55–65% of Maximum Heart Rate	Anaerobic Resistance Training	Stretching & Deep Breathing
Duration:	Duration:	Duration:	Duration:
5 to 10 minutes	*20 minutes*	*40 minutes*	*5 to 10 minutes*

Resistance training must always be preceded by warm-ups with stretching and aerobic exercise for at least 10 minutes. Cardiovascular workouts must always be preceded by stretching but do not necessarily have to be followed by resistance training, although this is ideal. Both aerobic and anaerobic exercise need to be followed by release of muscles through stretching and several deep breaths.

Exercise, Mood, and Behavior

People who exercise feel better and perform better, regardless of age or occupation. That's because exercise releases feel-good neurotransmitters, epinephrine and norepinephrine, plus painkilling endorphins. At the same time, exercise lowers the stress hormone cortisol. These changes lead to improved memory, better concentration, and a more positive outlook on life. And there's always the bonus of improved body image.

This might seem unimportant within the context of anti-aging, but it's extremely important to people of all ages. A group of 49 college women were enrolled in a strength-training class that met twice a week. The women were evaluated before beginning the class and again at the end of 12 weeks. Body weight and fat mass changed very little, but maximal lifting ability increased from 5 to 11 pounds. The women reported that they felt healthier, more fit, and had a better body shape and self-image.

Human data show that "executive functions" processed in the frontal lobe and brain hippocampus may be selectively maintained or even enhanced with higher levels of fitness. Recent evidence suggests that neuron development at least in the hippocampus may be increased by exercise. Nonneuronal tissues in the brain also seem to respond to exercise and learning stimulation. Exercise increases blood flow to the brain, causing release of nitric oxide, a powerful brain stimulant.

A team of researchers from Northern Arizona University in Flagstaff examined the effects of exercise duration on mood. A group of individuals were assessed for mood states after taking a short rest, then participating in one of three riding times—10, 20, or 30 minutes—on a stationary bicycle. Heart rate levels during exercise were controlled at 60 percent of maximum oxygen consumption levels. Significant improvement in vigor, with reduced levels of fatigue, confusion, and total negative mood occurred after 10 and 20 minutes of riding. No further improvements were found after 20 minutes. These observations indicate that shorter periods of exercise undertaken throughout the day result in positive fitness, mood and health benefits.

In a college study, 100 students were divided into two groups: one taking a semester swimming class and the other a semester fitness lecture class. Not surprisingly, swimmers reported significantly less tension, depression, anger, confusion, and more vigor after exercising than before. Moreover, it didn't matter whether the swimmers were beginners or intermediates, and there were no gender differences in the amount of mood change associated with swimming. However, the women reported significantly less tension, anxiety, depression, anger, and confusion than the men.

A study of 103 healthy middle-age women explored the association between fitness, displays of impulsive anger and neurotic anger, and lipid profile. The results showed that impulsive anger but not neurotic anger is a predictor of negative lipid profile including high total cholesterol and high LDL, high triglycerides, and increased levels of glucose. A negative lipid profile significantly increases the risk of cardiovascular heart disease. The physically fit women displayed less anger and did not have a negative lipid profile.

In a study of overweight or obese individuals with osteoarthritis of the knee, 32 participants were tested for pain relief following exercise. Although increased pain was reported immediately following exercise, it was significantly lower later in the day at a time when it was usually most intense. Exercise can help relieve osteoarthritis pain, even if patients don't lose weight. Obviously, losing weight could be expected to further relieve knee pain. That's why you need the Anti-Aging Solution 5-Step Plan as a complete road map for anti-aging.

CHAPTER 6

Step 4: Supplement Your Genes

Metabolic harmony requires an optimum intake of each micronutrient: deficiency distorts metabolism in numerous and complicated
ways, many of which may lead to DNA damage.
—Bruce Ames, Ph.D., Department of Molecular and Cell Biology,
University of California, Berkeley

We have established that your long-term health depends on making
specific adjustments in your menu plans, most notably reducing the
amount of food you eat and incorporating a wider range of brightly
colored foods. In chapter 4, we emphasized the healing power of foods
vis-à-vis phytonutrients that have anti-aging, DNA-protecting, and dis-
ease-preventing effects. The power of healing foods comes from their
broad-based ability to prevent disease by nutritionally fortifying the
biochemical processes that have been naturally selected by evolution
to protect us from disease and aging.

However, even with a dramatic change in diet, supplements containing concentrated forms of nutrients usually from food sources are
needed to overcome the damaging effects of micronutrient deficiencies,
pollution, radiation, and internally generated free radicals. Since vitamins and minerals are required to cofactor metabolic enzymes,
micronutrient deficiencies can cause profound alterations in normal
cellular function. Nutraceutical supplements can also amp up DNA

repair capability, the bottom line in preventing most diseases by reducing DNA damage.

Micronutrient Deficiency and DNA Damage

Approximately forty micronutrients are essential for normal metabolism. According to Dr. Bruce Ames, "Micronutrient deficiency can mimic radiation (or chemicals) in damaging DNA by causing single- and double-strand breaks, oxidative lesions, or both," which in turn are the root cause of most diseases. The table on the following page lists the most prevalent vitamin and mineral deficiencies, food sources for these vitamins and minerals, and the kind of DNA damage that occurs when they are deficient, resulting in deleterious effects.

Correcting micronutrient deficiencies requires doses higher than the recommended daily intake (RDI) to activate sluggish metabolic enzymes. Dr. Ames has estimated that about fifty human genetic diseases are due to defective enzymes and that supplying the appropriate coenzyme and/or cofactor in optimum doses can induce greater enzyme activity.

In addition to preventing or correcting DNA damage, other micronutrients are needed to activate enzymes involved in important metabolic pathways that are derailed in the aging process. Yet most multivitamin supplements, even those labeled as "anti-aging," are missing many of these key micronutrients and provide only the minimum RDI of vitamins and minerals needed to prevent aging conditions.

RDI Levels and Anti-aging Benefits

The Institute of Medicine, National Academy of Sciences, has established panels of experts to review micronutrient requirements. The panel reviews volumes of scientific evidence before making its recommendations on dietary intakes. The recommendations known as RDIs, which are familiar to you from reading the nutritional fact panels on foods and supplements, are given as a guideline for healthy people and are not necessarily absolute. The expert panels have recently began establishing optimum levels and upper limits for micronutrients. However, these are still based on the average healthy person eating an adequate diet and do not necessarily allow for anti-aging benefits. In fact, it has only recently been established within the scientific community that diet alone may not supply all the micronutrients needed to maintain good health.

DNA Damage and Conditions Stemming from Micronutrient Deficiencies

Micro-Nutrient	Food Sources	% People Deficient	Anti-Aging Daily Intake	DNA Damage from Deficiency	Conditions Stemming from Deficiency
Folic acid	Dark green veggies	10%	400–1,000 mcg	Chromosome breaks, base substitution Required for cytosine and thymidine synthesis	Colon cancer, cardiovascular disease, brain dysfunction, birth defects
Vitamin B_{12}	Meat	4% get less than half the RDI	400–600 mcg	Same as folic acid Required for all four bases	Nerve damage, breast cancer, plus same as folic acid
Vitamin B_6	Whole-grain bread, cereals	10% get less than half the RDI	50–100 mg	Same as folic acid Required for thymidine synthesis	Same as folic acid and B_{12}
Vitamin C	Fruits, vegetables, liver	15% get less than half the RDI	750–1,000 mg	Free radical (DNA oxidation) damage is similar to that from radiation	Cataract risk increased 4 times, cancer, cardiovascular disease
Vitamin E	Nuts, vegetable oils	20% get less than half the RDI	200–800 IU	Radiation mimic (DNA oxidation), damage is similar to radiation	Cancer: colon (↑2X), cardiovascular disease (↑1.5 X), immune dysfunction
Iron	Meat, fortified cereals	7% get less than half the RDI	9–18 mg	DNA breaks, radiation mimic	Brain dysfunction, immune dysfunction, cancer
Zinc	Meat, whole grains	18% get less than half the RDI	10–25 mg	Chromosome breaks, radiation mimic	Brain dysfunction, immune dysfunction, cancer
Niacin	Meat, legumes	2% get less than half the RDI	100–500 mg	Disables DNA repair enzymes (polyADP-ribose)	Neurological symptoms, memory loss

Note: 1 percent of the U.S. population = 2.7 million people in 1998. For percentages of the population listed for each micronutrient, with the exception of folic acid, intakes were less than half the recommended daily intake (RDI). Additional micronutrient deficiencies will likely be recognized as time passes.

Source: Adapted from Ames, B. *Toxicology Letters* 1998; /Vol.102–103:5–18.

While scientists estimate that poor diet contributes to about one-third of preventable cancers—on a par with smoking—optimizing vitamin and mineral intake with high-dose multivitamin and mineral supplements may prevent cancer and other chronic diseases. Scientists at the Cooper Institute in Dallas, Texas, found that multivitamins with strong antioxidant components not only raised blood levels of key nutrients but also reduced homocysteine and LDL cholesterol oxidation—two important risk factors in cardiovascular disease. Physicians do not routinely check blood levels of the key micronutrients that might reveal subclinical micronutrient deficiencies.

Subclinical Micronutrient Deficiencies

Epidemiologists at Harvard Medical School have identified several metabolic disorders that stem from suboptimal intakes of vitamins and minerals. Yet these disorders do not fit the classic definition of vitamin deficiency, and standard blood tests do not reveal such conditions. Consequently, physicians are reluctant to routinely recommend vitamin and mineral supplements as disease preventives. The Harvard scientists have stressed that supplements are not a substitute for a good diet with its wide diversity of phytonutrients but should be used as secondary therapy in treating metabolic disorders. Given the state of the art and being consistent with it, our anti-aging supplement plan recommends only nutrients aimed at specific molecular targets to correct aging conditions.

Zeroing in on Molecular Targets

Anti-aging supplements augment a healthy diet and reduce aging effects. We will show you how the following molecular targets are coordinated with the anti-aging supplement plan:

- Reducing oxidative stress with natural fat and water-soluble antioxidants
- Minimizing DNA, protein, carbohydrate, and lipid damage with lipoic acid, coenzyme Q-10, and N-acetyl-carnitine
- Enhancing DNA repair with CAE extract, nicotinamide, and zinc
- Improving immune function and blocking inflammation with CAE extract, aged garlic extract, medicinal mushrooms, probiotics, digestive enzymes, and herbs

- Optimizing gene expression within cells with fatty acids, B vitamins, minerals, vitamin A, and amino acids
- Balancing hormones with phytoestrogens, dehydroepiandrosterone (DHEA), and melatonin

Anti-Aging Nutraceutical Supplements

The anti-aging supplement plan contains specific nutraceuticals that everyone needs to prevent damage to genes, repair DNA, counter inflammation, and optimize gene expression. Although stress reduction, exercise, and diet all help balance hormones, specific supplements are also helpful. In chapter 7, you will learn about topical hormone balancing.

Nutraceutical is a term that was coined in the late 1980s by Stephen De Felice, M.D., to describe chemicals in foods that have medicinal power. Food phytochemicals are one class of nutraceuticals, and these were discussed in chapter 4. In this chapter, we present nutraceuticals that are taken as dietary supplements. They include vitamins, minerals, amino acids, herbs, and semivitamins that have been shown to have specific effects on genes and enzymatic processes.

Nutraceutical supplements are taken with each meal and are an important component of the Anti-Aging Solution, because it's virtually impossible to ensure an optimum intake of essential anti-aging nutrients from diet alone. The basic supplement plan applies to everyone. In some cases, additional amounts of a particular supplement may be recommended. For example, those who smoke need extra antioxidants.

The results from your home test kits as outlined in appendix A may suggest specific natural hormone replacement, either as topical or oral hormone precursors. Here are the specifics on the nutraceutical supplements.

Reducing Oxidative Stress

You learned about color-coded eating in chapter 4 and how the various colors indicate which phytochemicals are present. Most of these phytochemicals have powerful antioxidant properties. Our supplement plan enhances the antioxidant power of a colorful diet. Let's begin by discussing supplements from the yellow, orange, red group—the carotenoids.

Carotenoids

Over 600 different carotenoids with names spanning the alphabet have been identified. Among them are alpha-, beta-, gamma-, and delta-carotenes, astaxanthin, beta-cryptoxanthin, lutein, lycopene, phyto-fluene, and zeaxanthin. Beta-carotene has been the most studied of the carotenes, and for many years its importance was attributed to being a precursor of vitamin A. Recently it has been discovered that alpha- and gamma-carotene are also precursors of vitamin A. Furthermore, scientists believe the most important benefits of all the carotenoids are their antioxidant capacity and cell-signaling activities.

The antioxidant properties of the carotenoids have been the object of intense interest among scientists, because these fat-soluble phytonutrients with an affinity for membranes trap free radicals generated within the cell or attempting entry from the outside. A most remarkable attribute of carotenoids is their ability to regulate cell-to-cell communication, and this is the basis for many of their anti-cancer and immune-boosting effects.

Amazingly, carotenoids express a preference for protecting a particular type of membrane. Astaxanthin, lutein, and zeaxanthin protect the eyes; lycopene protects the prostate; beta-cryptoxanthin protects joints; and carotenes protect DNA. Astaxanthin and lycopene are most protective against radiation from ultraviolet A (UVA) and ultraviolet B (UVB). Following are some highlights from the scientific literature about the benefits of carotenoid supplements:

- Xanthophyll carotenoids, vitamins C and E can delay onset of macular degeneration and cataracts.
- Astaxanthin, canthaxantin, and beta-carotene have anti-cancer activity.
- High levels of carotenoids from supplements reduce oxidative damage to DNA.
- Carotenoids protect against free radicals.
- Astaxanthin and lycopene are more protective against UV radiation than beta-carotene.
- High serum levels of lycopene may play a role in the early prevention of atherosclerosis.
- Supplemental beta-cryptoxanthin and zinc reduce the risk of rheumatoid arthritis.
- Curcumin from turmeric scavenges nitric oxide, thus reducing inflammation and protecting against cancer.

Daily Prescription for Carotenoid Supplementation

Key: milligrams = mg, micrograms = mcg, international units = IU

1. Mixed natural carotenoids—5,000 to 10,000 IU of vitamin A activity from *Daniella salina*
2. Lycopene—2 to 5 mg from tomato seed extract
3. Lutein and zeaxanthin—2 to 5 mg from extract of marigold flowers
4. Turmeric rhizome *(Curcuma longa)* 95 percent extract—100 mg
5. Astaxanthin, algal source—1 to 10 mg

Note: The doses are appropriate for full-range carotenoid supplementation. Higher doses may be needed if individual carotenoids are selected for therapy.

Vitamin E

Vitamin E is unquestionably the best-known antioxidant and is the principal protective agent found in cellular membranes. Natural vitamin E is a combination of eight related compounds, each with slightly different activity. These include four tocopherols (alpha, beta, gamma, and delta) and four tocotrienols, also designated by the Greek letters.

Vitamin E scavenges free radicals attempting entry into cells or their organelles such as mitochondria. In the process of free radical destruction, vitamin E itself becomes a free radical called α-tocopheroxyl. This would have a devastating effect on cells if other members of the cellular antioxidant network, including vitamin C, alpha-lipoic acid, NADH, and coenzyme Q-10, were not present. These other antioxidants restore α-tocopheroxyl to fully reactive α-tocopherol. Consequently, when several are present in the diet or supplemented, less vitamin E is required. It was established in the 1980s that levels of vitamin E drop as we age, necessitating higher intake to achieve anti-aging benefits. The scientific evidence shows that vitamin E

- Lowers LDL cholesterol oxidation
- Reduces the risk of stroke by protecting LDL cholesterol
- Lowers the risk of heart disease
- Improves insulin action in healthy older individuals and those with diabetes
- Raises levels of glutathione, another antioxidant and detoxifying agent, in diabetic patients

- Protects against exercise-induced oxidative damage
- Slows the development of cataracts
- Reduces inflammation and enhances immune response
- Reduces cognitive decline in aging

Tocotrienols

Tocotrienols have anti-aging therapeutic activity beyond that of vitamin E. In fact, gamma-tocotrienol is the most potent cholesterol-lowering member of the entire E family. Recent studies have shown that tocotrienols

- Lower a number of lipid-related risk factors, including total cholesterol, LDL, apolipoprotein B, and lipoprotein A (gamma-tocotrienol 200 mg per day lowered cholesterol 31 percent)
- Suppress inflammatory agents such as thromboxane B2 and platelet factor 4
- Reduce blood levels of lipid peroxides
- Induce apoptosis and inhibit tumor growth in human breast cancer cells

Daily Prescription for Vitamin E and Tocotrienols
1. Vitamin E from natural mixed tocopherols—200 IU
2. Natural mixed tocotrienols—100 IU

Sulfur-Containing Antioxidants

Cruciferous vegetables contain a family of sulfur compounds known collectively as glucosinolates. Among them are diindolylmethane (DIM), sulforaphane, calcium D-glucarate, and indole-3-carbinol (I3C). They have been standardized in extracts of cruciferous vegetables and used in numerous trials that validate their anti-aging benefits.

- I3C induces detoxification enzymes that help prevent breast cancer.
- Indole and thiosulfonate compounds isolated from cruciferous vegetables may prevent DNA adducts and colon cancer.
- Isothiocyanates help prevent cancers of the lung, mammary gland, esophagus, liver, small intestine, colon, and bladder.
- Calcium D-glucarate favorably alters hormone response and may help prevent cancers of the breast, prostate, and colon.
- DIM induces apoptosis and confers protection against DNA damage.

- DIM protects against prostate, cervical, and colon cancer. It also has anti-androgenic effects.
- Aged garlic extract (AGE) inhibits TNFα and NF-κB, preventing damage to DNA and reducing inflammation.
- AGE helps prevent liver damage from acetaminophen.
- Supplementation with AGE reduces production of F_2 isoprostanes, which are by-products of oxidative damage.
- AGE reduces cholesterol and homocysteine levels, which are significant risk factors in cardiovascular disease.

Daily Prescription for Sulfur Compounds

1. Extract of cruciferous vegetables—500 to 1,000 mg (or for special needs, one of the individual actives as follows)
2. Calcium D-glucarate—500 mg for colon protection
3. I3C—250 mg for breast protection
4. DIM—150 mg for prostate protection
5. Garlic—100 mg for cardiovascular and immune protection

Vitamin C and Polyphenols

Vitamin C is a complex of ascorbate and related compounds that have antioxidant and anti-cancer effects. Natural vitamin C is much more than ascorbic acid, and to get the full benefit of the vitamin, the entire complex should be taken. This ensures effectiveness with much lower doses and fewer side effects such as gastrointestinal irritation. It also reduces the pro-oxidant effect of large doses of ascorbic acid, particularly in the presence of iron.

Ascorbate is the primary water-soluble antioxidant and a key player in the antioxidant network whereby oxidized vitamin E is regenerated (see details below). Ascorbate is the first line of defense against free radicals in body fluids.

- Vitamin C reduces cataract risk.
- A natural citrus extract of vitamin C is more bioavailable than ascorbic acid.
- Natural citrus extract of vitamin C may be a more vigorous free radical scavenger than vitamin E in preventing LDL cholesterol oxidation.
- Vitamin C along with selenium inhibits protein glycation and formation of advanced glycation end products.
- Flavonoids protect against several chronic diseases including

cardiovascular disease, cerebrovascular disease, lung and prostate cancers.

- Flavonoids can block prostate-specific antigen and aromatase, which are androgen-regulating proteins implicated in prostate cancer.
- Flavonoids block the cancer proliferative effects of xenoestrogens. They have anti-estrogenic and anti-cancer effects.
- Green tea catechins (EGCG) have potent anti-allergenic activity.
- Green tea catechins have thermogenic properties that aid weight loss.
- Grapeseed proanthocyanidin extract protects against DNA fragmentation and increased apoptotic cell death in oral keratinocytes of smokers.
- Pycnogenol is an effective anti-inflammatory agent.
- Resveratrol may activate anti-aging enzymes.
- Cranberry juice supplements reverse cholesterol transport, decreasing total cholesterol and LDL.

Daily Prescription for Vitamin C and Polyphenols
1. Natural vitamin C from citrus—500 to 1,000 mg
2. Mixed flavonoids—100 to 500 mg
3. Grapeseed proanthocyanidins or pycnogenol—10 to 50 mg
4. Resveratrol extract—2 to 20 mg
5. Green tea extract standardized for EGCG—50 to 100 mg
6. Cranberry juice extract—500 mg to prevent recurring urinary tract infections; 15 to 25 mg for antioxidant protection

Summary of Benefits from Antioxidant Combinations

A British team of researchers studied the connection between neurodegenerative diseases and antioxidant levels. The results were published in the *Monthly Journal of the Associations of Physicians* in 1999. Here is a summary of their findings:

- Alzheimer's patients had significantly lower levels of vitamins A, C, and E.
- Patients with vascular dementia had lower levels of vitamins A, C, and beta-carotene.
- Low levels of lycopene were associated with Parkinson's disease but not Alzheimer's or vascular dementia.
- No single antioxidant was universally low in these three conditions. This last finding underscores the importance of supplying

all of the antioxidants mentioned above in staving off neurodegenerative disorders.

Restoring blood levels of antioxidants may also do the following:

- TNFα, a promoter of inflammation and free radical damage, may be inhibited.
- Antioxidants superoxide dismutase, glutathione, catalase, and energy transporter carnitine may decrease the risk or severity of rheumatoid arthritis.
- Long-term use of vitamins E, C, and folic acid help maintain normal brain function as we age.
- Beta-carotene, flavonoids, vitamin C, and vitamin E may reduce the occurrence of Alzheimer's disease.
- Vitamins C and E from supplements reduce the risk of ovarian cancer.

Decreasing DNA Damage in Mitochondria

Oxidative damage to mitochondrial DNA is the root of aging and aging conditions. Among supplements, coenzyme Q_{10} (CoQ_{10}) and alpha-lipoic acid provide the most powerful protection for mitochondrial DNA.

Coenzyme Q_{10}

Ubiquinone or ubidecarenone is concentrated within mitochondria as part of the energy (ATP)-producing apparatus in these cellular power plants. It is generally understood that most aging conditions result from mitochondrial dysfunction due in part to insufficient CoQ_{10}, which works as an electron acceptor/proton donor in converting energy-rich molecules into ATP. Being vital to life, CoQ_{10} in several forms is found in all living species. Yet it has not been accorded vitamin status for humans because it can be synthesized within the body. It does require twelve other micronutrients including several B vitamins, vitamin C, and trace elements for its conversion from the amino acid tyrosine. Interestingly, the same micronutrients are required for the manufacture of DNA bases from tyrosine. Consequently, micronutrient deficiencies can lead to low levels of CoQ_{10}, requiring that it be supplemented along with its vitamin and mineral cofactors.

A major side effect of statin drugs such as Lovastatin is depletion of body stores of CoQ_{10}. Statins are used to reduce high cholesterol, a risk factor for cardiovascular disease. Paradoxically, low levels of CoQ_{10}

can weaken heart muscle and lead to cardiomyopathy. Therefore, CoQ_{10} must be supplemented when statin drugs are used.

There are two critical roles for CoQ_{10}—namely those of antioxidant and bioenergetic molecules—and these roles are interdependent. Stress reduces energy and can make you sick. It has been well established that stress increases oxidative burden, requiring greater amounts of antioxidants to protect cells. In this case, less antioxidants are available for energy production. At the same time, stress reduces the levels of micronutrients that are needed to step up internal production of CoQ_{10} to meet increased antioxidant demand. Additionally, CoQ_{10} levels drop as we age. Following are some scientific highlights on CoQ_{10}, which has been shown to

- Inhibit lipid oxidation in both cell membranes and low-density lipoproteins, and protect DNA from oxidative damage
- Protect exercising muscle from oxidative damage
- Prevent oxidative damage to the brain
- Stabilize membranes and reconstitute vitamin E as an antioxidant
- Enhance cardiac function and speed recovery from heart attack; effective as an adjunct therapy during cardiac surgery
- Maintain healthy apoptosis and may help prevent cancer
- Prevent thyroid disorders

L-Carnitine (N-Acetyl-L-Carnitine)

The energetic effects of CoQ_{10} are enhanced by supplementation with L-carnitine (N-acetyl-L-carnitine). Carnitine is considered a conditionally essential nutrient for mitochondrial energetics. Carnitine transports fatty acids across membranes so that they can be converted into energy. Since heart muscle relies on fatty acids as a source of fuel, conditional carnitine deficiency reduces heart function. Carnitine is synthesized within the body from amino acids, particularly S-adenosyl methionine and lysine, with vitamin B_6, niacin, iron, and ascorbate required for its synthesis. Consequently, carnitine deficiency may occur along with other micronutrient deficiencies. N-acetyl-L-carnitine can be considered the coenzyme form of the nutrient and is preferred for maintaining brain and nerve function during aging.

Alpha-Lipoic Acid

Alpha-lipoic acid is both water and lipid soluble, making it a universal antioxidant that provides protection throughout the body. Alpha-lipoic acid is an important member of the antioxidant network, restoring both water (vitamin C) and lipid-soluble (vitamin E, CoQ_{10}) antioxidants to full scavenging capacity. Lipoic acid can regenerate itself using a niacin coenzyme (NADH). Lipoic acid is also a vital coenzyme in the conversion of glucose to cellular energy, thus helping to maintain blood glucose balance.

Lipoic acid protects DNA by sequestering free radical–generating metals, and it has positive effects on gene expression. It is readily absorbed through the skin as well as the digestive system. You will read more about its topical application in chapter 7.

- Lipoic acid is an ideal antioxidant active in protecting both lipids and aqueous cellular components.
- Lipoic acid blocks NF-κB binding to DNA.
- Lipoic acid supplementation improves carbohydrate metabolism and reduces insulin resistance in muscles.
- Lipoic acid reduces harmful diabetic effects on red blood cell lipid membranes.
- Lipoic acid may reverse memory loss by reducing DNA/RNA oxidation.
- Lipoic acid increases brain energy and skeletal muscle performance.

Daily Prescription for CoQ_{10}, Carnitine, and Alpha-Lipoic Acid

1. CoQ_{10}—30 to 280 mg solubilized and water miscible (Q-gels) in soft gelatin capsules
2. L-carnitine fumerate or acetyl-L-carnitine—50 to 100 mg for general anti-aging benefits and as part of a comprehensive antioxidant supplement
3. Alpha-lipoic acid—500 to 1,000 mg for diabetes, diabetic complications, or to reduce advanced glycation end products

Note: When these energetic nutrients are combined, less of each is required.

Enhancing DNA Repair

The only known natural substance to enhance DNA repair is CAE and the combination of the micronutrients niacinamide, zinc, and carotenoids. This function is critical to slowing the aging process and reducing age-related conditions. Dr. Pero and his colleagues in the

Department of Biochemistry, University of Lund, Sweden, and other researchers have found that CAE extract

- Enhances immune function without toxicity
- Enhances antibody response to vaccination
- Induces apoptosis and slows growth of leukemic cells
- Enhances DNA repair with niacin, carotenes, and zinc
- Nonselectively increases immune cells

The five case studies below illustrate how CAEs can relieve aging conditions stemming from inflammation and lowered immune response.

Richard is 60 years old and had surgery to repair herniated disks. Following the surgery he was bothered by sciatica that had persisted for 8 years. He had tried several medications to relax his muscles and reduce inflammation, but none had worked. He began taking the extract containing CAEs (350 mg) twice a day. Soon after beginning the supplement, he noticed a great improvement in his flexibility and reduction in stiffness. As long as he took the supplement, he experienced no pain or sciatica. However, when he stopped, the symptoms returned. Once he began taking the supplement again, the pain and stiffness disappeared. Richard has also noticed an improved resistance to colds and flu.

Dan, a newly retired postal worker, found a pea-size lesion on the right side of his forehead. Within 6 months, it had grown to the size of a small egg. His physician advised surgery, but before it could be scheduled Dan began taking 350 mg of the water-soluble extract containing CAEs every day. The tumor began shrinking dramatically and Dan delayed the surgery. After 4 months, the tumor had all but disappeared, so surgery wasn't needed. Dan now takes a daily anti-aging multiple vitamin and mineral that includes CAEs as preventive therapy.

Rose is a 31-year-old marketing professional. She had been diagnosed with rheumatoid arthritis 12 years previously. Her condition had deteriorated, so she had been dependent on several medications for the past 2 years. These were extremely toxic medications—prednisone, the immune-suppressant drug Azulfadine, and Paquenil, an anti-arthritic drug. In addition, she received cortisone injections in her inflamed joints 3 or 4 times a year. Periodic flare-ups were so pain intense that they registered at the top of the pain index. Not surprisingly, Rose had severe lifestyle limitations including difficulty driving a car, working on the computer, exercising, and unbearable pain while traveling.

She began taking the CAE extract, 350 mg twice a day, and continued to do so for 1 year. During the year, her dependence on prednisone dropped from 200 mg/day to 7.5 mg/day. She also gradually reduced and finally discontinued all her other medications. Best of all, Rose reports her quality of life has improved dramatically. She is able to keep up with her job, has better mental function, and feels she has gotten her life back to pre-arthritis days.

Florence is a 70-year-old woman with rheumatoid arthritis and borderline systemic lupus erythematosus from which she has suffered for many years. Florence was in constant pain, lethargic, and fatigued most of the time. Her joints were swollen, misshapen, inflamed, and extremely painful. The immune-suppressing drugs she was taking left her with little ability to fight off frequent colds and flu, and she was developing glaucoma and macular degeneration.

Florence has been taking the CAE extract (350 mg twice daily) for 18 months. Shortly after starting the supplement, she noticed a dramatic decrease in pain and inflammation. She has not had a cold or flu since beginning supplementation. Her physician has not only noted a dramatic reduction in her symptoms but also an improvement in her eyes. The doctor attributes the latter improvement to reduction in her rheumatoid symptoms.

Harry is a 30-year-old retailer who has had ulcerative colitis for over 10 years with frequent cramping, diarrhea, and bleeding. A sigmoidoscopy exam revealed that he had ulcers extending 2 feet into his colon. His physician had prescribed 500 mg/day of sulfasalazine, but the dose had been repeatedly increased in order to overcome increasing inflammation. The situation was becoming progressively worse and Harry decided to seek an alternative treatment for his condition.

At first he took the CAE extract (200 mg/day) along with sulfasalazine. He noticed an almost immediate relief in his condition and a reduction in inflammatory flare-ups. Not only did his diarrhea stop but there was no longer blood in his stools. Two months after beginning the CAEs, Harry had a colonoscopy, which showed a much smaller area of inflammation. Harry continues to take CAEs along with a very small dose of sulfasalazine to keep his condition in check. He has more energy and a positive outlook on life.

Daily Prescription for Enhancing DNA Repair
1. CAE extract—350 mg
2. Niacinamide—100 to 300 mg
3. Zinc (amino acid chelated)—10 to 25 mg in addition to a balance of other amino acid–chelated minerals

Improving Immune Function and Blocking Inflammation

CAE Extract

Genetic damage alters the way your immune system works. Pro-inflammatory factors are increased while those that reduce inflammation are reduced. Consequently, blocking damage to DNA with antioxidants and enhancing its repair with CAEs reduces pro-inflammatory agents.

Dr. Pero and his colleagues have found that CAEs are thus effective anti-inflammatory agents, particularly with regard to gastrointestinal disorders such as irritable bowel syndrome, Crohn's disease, and other inflammatory conditions. NF-κB and elevated TNFα occupy pivotal roles in chronic inflammation and cancer progression. They also interfere with chemotherapeutic treatment for cancer. C-Med blocks NF-κB, in turn reducing TNFα and restoring apoptosis.

- NF-κB inhibition is a new target for treating asthma.
- TNFα contributes to airway obstruction in asthma.
- Niacinamide has anti-inflammatory effects.
- A water-soluble extract containing CAEs reduces inflammation by inhibiting NF-κB.
- Chemotherapy may be enhanced by reducing NF-κB–blocked apoptosis

Medicinal Mushrooms

Medicinal mushrooms contain phytochemicals that help reduce the effects of stress on your body and support immune function. They belong to a class of nutraceuticals known as *adaptogens* because they help the body restore homeostasis during stressful times. There are three important attributes of adaptogens:

1. They do not cause harm and do not place additional stress on the body.
2. They help the body adapt to various environmental and biological stressors.
3. They have nonspecific action, supporting all organ and regulatory systems in the body.

Several polysaccharides, lectins, and terpenoids have been isolated from fungi and studied for their adaptogenic and immune-potentiating effects. Among the most familiar mushrooms are shiitake *(Lentinus edodes)*, reishi *(Ganoderma lucidum)*, cordyceps *(Cordyceps sinensis)*, and maitake *(Grifola frondosa)*. Several lesser-known ones are turkey tail *(Trametes versicolor)*, split gill *(Schizophyllum commune)*, mulberry yellow polypore *(Phellinus linteus)*, and cinder conk *(Inonotus obliquus)*. Cordyceps has been known in China for at least 1,000 years as the anti-aging mushroom and reishi is considered sacred.

The only medicinal mushroom you'll find in the grocery store is shiitake, which makes an excellent addition to soups and other combination dishes, especially when your immune system is challenged. Maitake can be harvested from the wild but isn't sold in stores. All mushrooms are good for you, but culinary mushrooms are weak therapeutically as compared to medicinal mushrooms, which have a long history of use in Asia and are becoming increasingly popular in Western societies. Additionally, an active polysaccharide called beta-1,3-glucan has been isolated from yeast *(Saccharomyces* species) and is available as an immune-enhancing supplement. Here is a brief summary of published studies on medicinal mushrooms and beta glucans:

- Mushroom polysaccharides have remarkable anti-tumor activity.
- Mushrooms have anti-hyperlipidemic, hypotensive, and hypoglycemic actions.
- Beta-glucan from maitake mushrooms may induce apoptosis in prostate cancer cells.
- Shiitake extracts have reduced cholesterol and have anti-viral effects.
- Mushrooms are high fiber and function as prebiotics, antioxidants, and antibiotics.

A case study involving seven men and seven women with an average age of 60 years showed remarkable results when CAEs were combined with an extract containing several medicinal mushrooms. This was a particularly interesting study because members of the study group noted dramatic improvement in several inflammatory conditions including allergies, pain with sleep loss, cardiovascular disease, and arthritis. The group was also tested for genetic damage and DNA repair capacity.

After only 4 weeks, DNA damage had been reduced—in some people by half—and DNA repair capacity was increased by an average of 18 percent. Pain was reduced 35 percent while fatigue dropped 21 percent. There was also an improvement in allergic reactions, with 7 percent less occurrence of skin rash. Surprisingly, all but one reported weight loss—an unexpected benefit. These were basically healthy people who had been taking a multivitamin and mineral formula, with some also taking medications. We will now discuss the results from two women in this study because their cases were especially dramatic.

> Mary was a 62-year-old who had suffered from rheumatoid arthritis for 17 years. She had been on a variety of medications with marginal results. Her main complaints were low energy, constant pain, and inability to sleep. After taking a combination of CAEs and mixed mushroom extracts for 4 weeks, she reported near complete recovery and exceptional energy, and she lost 15 pounds. She was absolutely delighted with her improvement, and her condition had continued to improve at last interview, even though she was no longer taking the CAE and mushroom extracts.

> Another 62-year-old woman named Fern had been suffering for 15 years from an inflammatory disorder that pinched the nerve passing from her lower leg into her foot. The condition is known as tarsal tunnel syndrome and involves severe pain, burning, and tingling in the soles of the feet. Fern could relieve the pain with massage and elevating her feet, but as soon as she moved, the pain was excruciating and worsened as the day advanced. Special shoe inserts brought some relief, but Fran depended on nonsteroidal anti-inflammatory drugs (NSAIDs) and steroid injections to help diminish the pain.
>
> She began taking CAE and medicinal mushroom extracts for 4 weeks as part of the group study. She was amazed to find that not only was she free of foot pain for the first time in her life but

her energy level was incredible. She also lost 5 pounds. She found that she was virtually pain-free and only needed to take NSAIDs occasionally.

Daily Prescription for Reducing Inflammation and Boosting Immunity

1. CAE extract—700 mg per day for 1 month, then maintain on 350 mg for medical conditions
2. Medicinal mushroom extracts—500 to 1,000 mg

Optimizing Gene Expression

Over the past few years, it has been documented that nutraceuticals directly influence gene expression, meaning they can activate or turn on certain genes while silencing or deactivating others. This has a direct effect on how the genetic code is expressed. Fatty acids are an important class of nutraceuticals that directly affect gene expression at the membrane surface.

The typical Western diet, with its emphasis on animal, cereal, and grain products, contains an unhealthy high ratio of omega-6 to omega-3 fatty acids. Fish and dark green vegetables are good sources of omega-3s and help keep the two fats in balance. Since dietary fat regulates gene expression, intake of the wrong fatty acids leads to changes in carbohydrate and lipid metabolism.

For many years, scientists focused on the role of hormones as regulators of gene expression; the role of fatty acids didn't emerge until much later. Hormones rely on specific receptors for uptake that are embedded in the membrane lipid bilayer. Any distortion of membrane architecture due to unavailability of the correct fatty acids affects hormone binding and alters gene expression within the cell. In this way, fatty acids can interfere with hormone regulation of a specific gene without having a generalized effect on overall hormonal control.

Fatty Acid Supplements

From an anti-aging perspective, fatty acids alter metabolism, change cellular response, and affect cellular growth and differentiation. These effects can be either beneficial or detrimental to the aging process. For example, omega-3-mediated suppression of serum triglycerides is beneficial, whereas omega-6-mediated promotion of insulin resistance is detrimental. The anti-aging benefits of fatty acids are

- Fatty acids modulate genetic expression of key metabolic enzymes.
- Polyunsaturated fatty acids and vitamin E reduce DNA damage.

As you learned in chapter 2, fatty acids make up the lipid bilayer of membranes, and oxidative damage to these lipids causes a dramatic change in cell function including cell differentiation, growth, cytokine adhesion molecule release, and eicosanoid production (anti- or pro-inflammatory). Listed here are nutrients that are particularly effective in stabilizing cell membranes.

- Fish oil supplements reduced the need for nonsteroidal anti-inflammatory drug (NSAID) use among patients with rheumatoid arthritis.
- DHA and fish oil supplements lower triglyceride levels.
- Fish oil supplements are effective in the treatment of atherosclerosis, thrombosis and embolic events, high triglycerides, hypertension, autoimmune disease, and allergic problems.
- Omega-3 fatty acid supplements reduce the risk of cardiovascular disease and sudden death in both men and women.

Daily Prescription for Fatty Acid Supplements

1. Fish oils—super omega-3s (EPA, 300 mg; DHA, 200 mg), 3 caps for cardiovascular and immune benefits
2. Fish or algal oils—high DHA, 500 mg for brain and nerve function, 1 to 2 caps
3. Gamma-linolenic acid (GLA)—200 to 600 mg from evening primrose or black currant oils for allergies and autoimmune conditions
4. Essential fatty acid combination—omega-3,6,9; 1,000 to 3,000 mg for general anti-aging benefits including dry skin, brittle nails, and thinning hair

B Vitamins

Nine B vitamins are considered essential for human nutrition: thiamine (B_1), riboflavin (B_2), niacin (B_3), pantothenic acid (B_5), pyridoxine (B_6), folic acid (B_9), cobalamin (B_{12}), biotin, and choline. Two others, inositol and para-aminobenzoic acid, are often included in supplement formulas. It is important to supplement all of the essential B vitamins because they cofactor enzymatic reactions in groups. However, it isn't necessary to supplement them in the same amount. As noted in the beginning of this chapter, niacin, folic acid, cobalamin, and pyridoxine are the most important in protecting DNA. However, the other B vitamins are just as important because they play vital roles in gene expression and cellular metabolism.

B vitamins are water soluble and are rapidly flushed from the system, so it is necessary to supply them daily. It isn't necessary to megadose, but it is important to get a balance of the entire B complex, preferably above the RDI. In some instances, higher doses of individual Bs may be required to overcome specific deficiencies. Optimum amounts of each B vitamin are given in the summary table of anti-aging supplements at the end of the chapter. Now let's look at the scientific overview for B vitamins:

- Nicotinamide (niacinamide) reverses aging mechanisms through possible modulation of histone acetylation.
- Niacin deficiency increases tumor incidence in the rat.
- Niacin supplementation increases DNA repair enzymes and helps overcome chemotherapy-induced damage.
- Vitamin and trace mineral supplements boost immunity in the elderly.
- B vitamins improve vascular function.
- Folate and vitamin B6 may be chemopreventive against breast cancer, particularly alcohol-related breast cancer.
- Folic acid may protect against colon cancer.
- Folic acid, B_{12}, and B_6 may lower homocysteine levels, a risk factor for cardiovascular disease.
- Folic acid may protect against Alzheimer's disease.
- Vitamin B_{12} may help resist HIV disease progression.
- Choline as alpha-glycerylphosphorylcholine (alpha-GPC) enhances overall brain function in young and older subjects.
- Alpha-GPC plays an important role in production of certain hormones and neurotransmitters such as acetylcholine and human growth hormone.

Daily Prescription for B Vitamins

1. B_1, B_2, and B_6—10 to 100 mg taken twice daily—morning and evening in divided doses
2. Niacin (B_3)—up to 300 mg taken as niacinamide or flush-free niacin, which does not cause the common niacin response of skin reddening and itching

3. Pantothenic acid (B_5)—up to 1,000 mg for lipid disorders and stress
4. Folic acid—400 to 800 mcg
5. B_{12} and biotin—150 to 300 mcg
6. Alpha-GPC—1,000 to 1,200 mg for cognition enhancement and growth hormone release

Minerals

Minerals function as cofactors for thousands of different metabolic enzymes. Zinc cofactors over 300 enzymatic reactions including those involved in DNA repair. Calcium, phosphorus, magnesium, and several trace minerals form skeletal structures. Calcium also has an important role in membrane transport and magnesium drives energy-producing reactions.

Minerals should always be taken together because there is the potential for depletion between competing minerals. For example, magnesium should always be taken with calcium in order to improve calcium utilization and guard against magnesium depletion. The best supplemental form of minerals to take are those bound to amino acids or small peptides, which escort minerals across the intestinal barrier and into the blood.

A promising area of investigation is the role of peptides as chaperones for guiding minerals to their reactive site. The discovery that peptide chaperones not only guide protein folding but also guide proteins to where they are needed earned the Nobel prize in medicine for Rockefeller University's Günter Blobel, M.D., in 1999. Other scientists have shown that this same protein chaperone system guides minerals to the correct reactive site and that this system is common among yeast, plant, and animal cells. Consequently, minerals such as selenium, copper, iron, and zinc that are bound to yeast chaperones appear to be highly bioavailable in humans. Here is an overview of the latest published studies on minerals:

- Calcium and vitamin D supplements reduce tooth loss.
- Calcium supplements improve lipid profiles in postmenopausal women.
- Calcium reduces the risk of colon cancer.
- Diabetes is a significant cause of low magnesium, which may lead to loss of appetite.

- Magnesium malate may provide energy reserves in fibromyalgia.
- Copper and zinc supplements may reduce bone loss in post-menopausal women.
- Zinc histidinate supplements are better absorbed than zinc sulfate.
- Chromium supplements are associated with reduced insulin resistance.

Daily Prescription for Minerals

1. Calcium citrate malate chelate—500 to 1,000 mg
2. Magnesium amino acid chelate—400 to 1,000 mg
3. Zinc histidinate, glycinate, or yeast bound—10 to 25 mg
4. Selenium monomethionate or yeast bound—200 mcg
5. Chromium polynicotinate or yeast bound—200 mcg
6. Manganese amino acid chelate—5 to 10 mg
7. Iodine from potassium iodate or kelp—150 mcg
8. Potassium amino acid complex—99 mg
9. Molybdenum amino acid chelate—50 to 150 mcg
10. Vanadium amino acid complex—50 to 100 mcg
11. Boron amino acid complex—1 to 3 mg

Prescription Summary

Let's summarize what a comprehensive anti-aging multivitamin and mineral combination should contain. The suggested supplements are available in anti-aging formulas that contain many of the extras that are considered important for a comprehensive anti-aging program.

Top-notch formulas that contain amino acid–chelated minerals in levels close to the RDI will require 6 to 8 tablets or capsules that are taken 2 to 3 times a day. The reason for so many pills is that minerals, particularly calcium and magnesium, are required in large doses. Minerals also require great amounts of amino acids to properly chelate them. In the case of calcium and magnesium, the ratio of amino acid to mineral is approximately 4:1. This means that 200 mg of magnesium will require 1,000 mg of magnesium amino acid chelate. The average capsule only holds 750 mg. Specialized multiple formulas or packets with anti-aging nutraceuticals require 4 capsules or tablets to be taken 3 times a day.

THE ANTI-AGING DAILY MULTIPLE SUPPLEMENT

Nutraceutical	Daily Amounts
Antioxidants to Decrease DNA Damage and Oxidative Stress	
Vitamin A	2,500–5,000 IU
Natural carotene mix (alpha-, beta-, and gamma-carotenes, yielding vitamin A activity) plus lutein, zeaxanthin, lycopene, and astaxanthin	5,000–10,000 IU
Vitamin E, blend of natural tocopherols and tocotrienols	200–400 IU
Vitamin K	50–400 mg
Vitamin D	200–400 IU
Vitamin C (natural citrus extract, ascorbyl palmitate, and ascorbate)	500–1,000 mg
Botanical antioxidants (green tea, garlic, bioflavonoids, anthocyanins, resveratrol, quercetin, and chrysin)	100–200 mg
DNA Repair and Reducing Inflammation	
CAE extract (this may require a separate supplement)	350 mg
Zinc histidinate or glycinate	10–25 mg
Niacinamide	100 mg up to 300 mg
Optimizing Gene Expression	
Vitamins B_1, B_2, and B_6	10–100 mg each
Pantothenic acid	Up to 1,000 mg
Folic acid	400–800 mcg
Vitamin B_{12} and biotin	150–300 mcg each
Calcium citrate and malate chelate	500–1,000 mg
Iodine (potassium iodate or kelp)	150 mcg
Magnesium amino acid chelate	400–1,000 mg
Zinc histidinate or glycinate (listed above)	10–25 mg
Selenium monomethionate	100–200 mcg
Copper amino acid chelate	0.5–2 mg
Manganese amino acid chelate	5–10 mg

Nutraceutical	Daily Amounts
Chromium amino acid chelate or polynicotinate	100–200 mcg
Molybdenum amino acid chelate	50–150 mcg
Potassium amino acid complex	99 mg
Boron amino acid chelate	1–3 mg
Vanadium amino acid chelate	50–100 mcg

The anti-aging multiple is for everyone. Depending on the results of your gene SNP screening test described in appendix A, you may need additional amounts of some supplements for your personal anti-aging program. In addition, the following nutraceuticals may be found in anti-aging formulas such as Optigene or others that are contained in a packet.

MITOCHONDRIAL ANTIOXIDANTS

CoQ_{10} (solubilized, Q-Gel)	60–120 mg
α-lipoic acid	50–100 mg
L-carnitine or N-acetyl-carnitine	50–100 mg

These antioxidants are essential for preserving mitochondrial function as we age. They are protective of the cardiovascular system (angina, hypertension, vascular and heart disease) and must be supplemented by those taking statin medications as already discussed. Alpha-lipoic acid and CoQ_{10} supplements are also indicated for prevention of protein glycation, oxidative stress, and diabetes. Natural synergism exists between L-carnitine and CoQ_{10} that increases the benefits when they are taken together. You will find these antioxidants in combinations as listed.

SULFUR ANTIOXIDANTS

Cruciferous vegetable extract	500–1,000 mg
Calcium D-glucarate	500 mg
Diindolylmethane (DIM)	150 mg
Aged garlic extract	100–500 mg

Sulfur antioxidants alter gene expression by blocking enzymes that promote tumors. Their activity is enhanced by vitamin C and some flavonoids. Certain extracts from cruciferous vegetables have specific protective effects. Garlic has anti-viral and anti-bacterial properties.

Enhancing Immune Function

Other anti-aging nutraceuticals such as probiotics (acidophilus), prebiotics (arabinogalactans or fructooligosaccharides), amino acids, and herbs may be included in the formula.

IMMUNE ENHANCERS

Digestive enzyme blend, pancreatin (8× concentration), or fungal enzymes	300–500 mg
Acidophilus blend (probiotic) minimum	3 billion units
Arabinogalactans *(Larix occidentalis)* or fructooli gosaccharides (FOS) (prebiotic)	200–500 mg
Medicinal mushrooms	500–1,000 mg

Blocking Inflammation

CAE extract is the primary nutraceutical for blocking inflammation because it inhibits NF-κB. Boswellin and curcumin are two popular Indian herbs that inhibit the pro-inflammatory COX-2 mediator. They have a long history of relieving joint inflammation and enhancing the anti-inflammatory effects of CAEs. Boswellin is available as a topical cream, and both herbs are available in capsules.

ANTI-INFLAMMATORY HERBS

Boswellin *(Boswellia serrata)* 70% extract capsules	200 mg 3 times daily
Boswellin cream 5% with capsaicin or methyl salicylate	3 times daily
Curcumin *(Curcuma longa)* 95% extract capsules	250 mg 3 times daily

Optimizing Gene Expression

Fatty acid supplements are also part of your anti-aging prescription; however, they are not included in multiple formulas such as the one described above, because they are oils and require soft gel encapsulation.

You will find a fatty acid capsule in many anti-aging formulas contained in packets. Spectrum Essential Oils offers a liquid formula that provides essential fatty acids you can take on a teaspoon or add to beverages or food.

We suggest four different formulas here. The fish oil omega-3 blend of EPA and DHA is for cardiovascular protection. The second omega-3 blend is for brain, nerve, and eye function. The blend of omega 3,6,9 is for general fatty acid supplementation. Gamma-linolenic acid (GLA), an omega-6 fatty acid, is recommended for allergies, rhinitis, or eczema.

GENE EXPRESSION

Fish omega-3 blend of EPA (300 mg), DHA (200 mg)	1,000–3,000 mg
Omega-3 blend of EPA (200 mg), DHA (500 mg), or Omega-3 DHA alone	500–1,000 mg 500 mg.
Omega-3,6,9 blend from flax, borage seed oils	1,000–3,000 mg
Omega-6 GLA from evening primrose or borage oil	200–600 mg

As you learned in chapter 2, certain segments of your genes are masked at the various stages of your life. However, overmethylation can silence genes that should be expressed. Consequently, methylating agents can help demethylate these vital sections of DNA and allow proper expression of the information they contain. Some of the most effective methylating agents are already included in our optimum multiple vitamin and mineral. These are vitamin B_{12} and folic acid. Other important methylating agents are listed below.

METHYLATING AGENTS

Alpha-GPC (glycerylphosphocholine) or choline	Up to 1,000 mg
S-adenosyl methionine (SAMe)	200–1,200 mg
Trimethylglycine (TMG)	100–200 mg
Dimethyaminoethanol (DMAE)	500–1,500 mg

These nutrients improve cognitive function, memory, and mental acuity and are often found in brain enhancement and mood-stabilizing formulas.

Hormones as Molecular Targets

Each step of the 5-Step Plan involves hormones, emphasizing the importance of balancing these cellular and metabolic regulators. Step 1 involves reducing cortisol levels through stress control. Step 2 balances cortisol and insulin through dietary change. Step 3 balances hormones through exercise, and step 4 balances hormones by optimizing the nutrients that catalyze the enzymatic reactions regulated by hormones. Now we will move on to the fifth and last step, which balances hormones with the goal of fine-tuning body composition and improving skin quality.

CHAPTER 7

Step 5: Make Over Your Skin and Body

What is more important in life than our bodies or in the world than what we look like?

—George Santayana

In this chapter, we will make two important connections in the Anti-Aging Solution. The first is that hormones, as regulators of your physical and emotional well-being, affect the appearance and function of your skin. The second is that your skin is the ideal vehicle for delivering gene-repairing, -balancing, and -healing nutrients into your body.

You will be presented with groundbreaking new information on how applying topical cosmeceutical agents including CAE extract and hormones can repair your genes and help reestablish internal organ homeostasis. You will see amazing results in your skin and body contours from this topical body lift approach. Alice's story best illustrates how this happens.

> I was taking prescribed synthetic hormone replacement therapy for several years and wanted a safe alternative. I knew there was a difference between synthetic and natural hormones, and I was alarmed about the health risks by continuing to take the synthetic hormones as long-term therapy. If I had been aware of the natural hormones, I would have never started the synthetic ones.
>
> I had started hormone replacement in the first place because I

wanted a healthier lifestyle and protection against heart disease and osteoporosis. Although I was worried about taking synthetic hormones, I felt I needed them to control menopausal symptoms such as night sweats, hot flashes, vaginal dryness, and mood swings.

When Dr. Giampapa first tested me, my estrogen levels were extremely high—way above the normal range. He immediately took me off the synthetic hormones and prescribed natural hormone cream containing estrogen, progesterone, DHEA, and testosterone. Since starting use of the cream, my hormone levels have tested in the normal range and I feel like a new person.

For my face, Dr. Giampapa recommended an anti-aging face cream with antioxidants and natural estrogen. He supported the topical therapy with an anti-aging vitamin formula along with dietary change—less carbohydrates and more protein, especially at dinner. Additionally he recommended an evening drink mix to increase growth hormone release and insulin-like growth factor while I slept.

Since starting the program 4 years ago, I have noticed numerous improvements in my quality of life—sleeping more soundly and not waking as often during the night. I also have improved memory and mood, and lower body fat. My energy level has improved dramatically—no midday slump. The skin on my face is tight and better toned and my hair is shiny again! My digestive system has improved thanks to the probiotics and digestive enzymes in the comprehensive anti-aging formula.

Alice's experience best illustrates the concept that anti-aging therapy is an inside/outside approach. The balanced organ function that Alice is enjoying is a result of outside application of antioxidants and hormones. But it's also due to the oral supplementation of vitamins, minerals, the special CAE extract, probiotics (acidophilus) and digestive enzymes that provide her cells with the proper nutritional environment to function optimally. Her face and body makeover is a remarkable testament to the power of this approach.

We also need to make clear that estrogen is actually three closely related compounds, all of which may be needed to achieve proper balance. Synthetic estrogen contains only the most toxic form and does not balance out the other forms, particularly estrone, the one that dominates after menopause. There will be further discussion on the differences between natural and synthetic hormones later in this chapter.

Let's now move onto a more detailed explanation of the skin in order to better appreciate how it functions to deliver vital nutrients and hormones to underlying tissues.

Your skin is the largest organ in your body. It protects you against chemical and microbe invasion and is the chief vehicle for eliminating toxins and body heat. Skin is also a protective barrier against moisture, heat, and dryness. Your skin receives and processes sensations such as heat, cold, and pressure. Peptides and neurohormones in your skin communicate this information to the central nervous system, which then frames an appropriate response. Your skin also plays a role in hormone production, producing vitamin D_3 (cholecalciferol) from sunlight (UVB). The vitamin is processed by the liver, then converted by the kidneys into the active hormone that increases intestinal uptake of calcium and phosphorus.

Hormones and Your Skin

Hormones generated within your body such as cortisol, insulin, and sex hormones also have a profound impact on the function of your skin and its appearance. Of the many hormones you produce, cortisol has the most profound effect on the appearance of your face and body.

Cortisol is directly related to a breakdown in skin collagen and elastin, as well as joint, bone, and muscle tissue. It also raises insulin levels, leading to glucose intolerance, which increases the deleterious effects of sugar on your skin.

Cortisol and insulin cause fat deposits around your middle (apple shape) and increase your waist to hip ratio (WHR). Refer to chapter 1 for the implications of WHR. Cortisol also reduces levels of youthful hormones (estrogens, progesterone, growth hormone, testosterone, and DHEA), causing fat deposits on your hips, thighs, breasts, buttocks, and arms. At the same time, your skin tone begins to relax, leading to flabbiness that's associated with aging.

Cortisol isn't the only hormone that affects your face and body. Other hormones affect the shape of your body and the fine lines you see in the mirror. There are two important concepts to keep in mind when thinking of hormones and their action. The first is communication and the second is homeostasis, the ability of the body to maintain balance within and in harmony with the environment. Organ systems throughout the body communicate with each other through a web-like model using signals controlled by hormones.

Communication

Intracellular communication is dependent on the level of hormones circulating in body fluids and their interaction with specific receptors anchored in the cell membrane. Hormones act directly on membrane receptors as well as other key molecules known as *second messengers* within the cell. Scientists call this communication signal transduction, and the effects are expressed throughout the cell. The cellular response of hormones involves receptors on genes and uptake of specific biomolecules that bind to DNA, resulting in modification of genetic expression.

The hypothalamus, the center of emotional, neurological, and physical connection, sits just above the pituitary gland. The pituitary is located in the center of your brain right behind your eyes. The hypothalamus acts as a rheostat, registering levels of circulating hormones, monitoring their effects, and initiating signals to regulate the hormone milieu. The hypothalamus signals the pituitary gland, causing it to release an activating hormone that travels to a target organ, which then secretes the specified hormone.

The parent molecule of all steroid hormones is cholesterol, which contains the basic steroid molecule. Each hormone eventually travels back to the hypothalamus, which then acts to either increase or decrease circulating levels of each hormone. This system is known as *feedback control.* It is an efficient system for maintaining hormone balance and homeostasis.

We depend on feedback control to regulate the use of natural hormones recommended in the Anti-Aging Solution. It allows the body to utilize the natural hormones for balancing by converting them into various forms. Hormones are part of the endocrine system.

As we have seen, hormones are messengers that coordinate communication between the various body systems including immune, nervous, gastrointestinal, skeletal, and endocrine. The endocrine system itself is a network made up of hormones, glands that secrete them, and their membrane receptors. Endocrine glands are unique in that they secrete hormones directly into the bloodstream. Each hormone is thus able to travel throughout the body, seeking its specific receptor on the cell surface of target organs.

Other glands, known as *exocrine glands,* deliver their secretions a short distance through tubes or ducts to targeted areas in the body. For example, the exocrine glands in your digestive system secrete digestive juices into nearby organs such as the stomach and intestines. Exocrine glands in your skin secrete oils that lubricate it. Hormone changes as we age have a profound effect on our skin, which we experience as dryness and thinning.

Having evolved over millions of years, hormones are responsible for integrating and maintaining optimum balance between organ systems. This internal balance, known as homeostasis, is the second major function of hormones.

Homeostasis

The degree of homeostasis you are experiencing at any given time determines your level of health and how quickly you are aging. As you age, hormone levels naturally decline, requiring an adjustment in hormone balance in order to maintain homeostasis. For example, the symptoms of menopause and andropause, the male equivalent of change of life, occur precisely because homeostasis hasn't reestablished following the normal drop in hormone levels that occur with aging. Consequently, your skin and body makeover includes testing your saliva for hormones, part of the home test kit we describe in appendix A, and natural topical hormone replacement. It also includes use of foods and supplements that help reestablish homeostasis.

Hormones and Their Target Organs

Most of us think of hormones within the context of reproduction. And while hormones such as estrogens, progesterone, and testosterone do regulate our sexual maturation and function, they are active throughout the body and are part of a vast system of communication. Thus, when levels of these hormones decrease, as we grow older, we experience changes in cognitive function, immune response, and sexual activity. It's important to understand that the changes we note as hormone levels decline are not due to reproductive hormones alone but altered communication throughout the entire network.

There are three groups of steroid hormones: (1) sex steroids, namely estrogen, testosterone, and androgens; (2) adrenal steroids, namely mineral corticoids and cortisol; (3) neurosteroids. These three groups of hormones interact with and affect those within the other groups. All three groups of hormones are active in the brain as well as in the body. Considerable evidence has shown that progesterone and the gonadal hormones testosterone and estrogens are neuroactive steroids that provide protection for the brain. Progesterone interacts with the neurotransmitters dopamine and acetylcholine, playing an important role in cognitive function. Progesterone also triggers characteristic responses associated with sexual behavior. In animals it initiates the *lordosis response,* a behavior that signals a female is receptive to mating. Furthermore, these neuroactive steroids may influence regeneration of peripheral motor neurons. Progesterone is synthesized in the nervous system by neurons and glial cells and plays a role in influencing gene expression in neurons.

While hormones are active throughout the body, they are regulated by the brain and central nervous system. Nature has provided for a smooth transition as hormone levels rise and fall. However, modern lifestyle and environmental agents create imbalances within the endocrine system and disrupt hormone function.

Endocrine Disrupters

Environmental contaminants that affect hormones in both men and women are called endocrine disrupters. According to Theo Colborn of the World Wildlife Fund in Washington, DC,

> Endocrine-disrupting chemicals can undermine neurological and behavioral development and subsequent potential of individuals exposed in the womb. . . . It may be expressed as reduced intellectual capacity and social adaptability, as impaired responsiveness to environmental demands, or in a variety of other functional guises. Widespread loss of this nature can change the character of human societies or destabilize wildlife populations.

Endocrine-disrupting agents are having a profound and dangerous effect on wildlife and human populations. These agents are found in fertilizers, plastics, herbicides, dioxin, phthalates, and wood and carpet materials.

Dangerous Chemicals

In two *Science News* reports published in 2000, senior environmental editor Janet Raloff reported on the dangers of a family of insidious chemicals called phthalates. These appear to affect male sexual development. Male fetuses exposed to phthalates in the first trimester of pregnancy may develop abnormal sexual organs. Some scientists worry that even babies and toddlers exposed to phthalates may have their sexual development altered. Phthalates are ubiquitous in plastics such as bags, food packaging, containers, and children's plastic toys. Phthalates are commonly used to make rigid polymers like plastic more flexible. They are also found in glues and solvents.

Phthalates are associated with precocious puberty in young girls. Extremely high levels have been found in the serum of girls with premature breast development. Fetal and childhood exposure to phthalates may also be a significant factor in the lower age at which puberty is occurring in girls in the United States.

Phthalates and other endocrine disrupters have been found in baby food and formulas, thus exposing children during the most vulnerable stage of their development. Cologne, fingernail polish, and dyes may be significant sources of contamination. You can reduce continued exposure to endocrine disrupters by reducing use of plastics in storing and cooking food. Avoid chemical sprays whenever possible and wear protective clothing during times of exposure. Read labels on products you commonly use to make sure they don't contain phthalates.

In addition to phthalates, DDT (dichlorodiphenyltrichloroethane; now banned in most countries), PCB (polychlorinated biphenyl), and certain pesticides are implicated in abnormalities of male fetal development. In men, these same chemicals have been blamed for testicular digenesis syndrome, a complex of disorders that include infertility stemming from poor semen quality, and rising levels of testicular and prostate cancers.

Scientists in Belgium did an interesting study in which they compared testosterone levels and sperm quality in 101 men from two cities: one outside Antwerp and another named Peer located in an agricultural belt. The men from Peer had significantly lower testosterone levels and sperm counts than those living closer to Antwerp. The greater exposure to agricultural chemicals, many of them endocrine disrupters, had a major impact on sexual function among men living in Peer.

Xenoestrogens are a specific class of endocrine disrupters that mimic the hormone estrogen. Some are found in plastics and pesticides such as DDT, heptachlor, and atrazine. Others come from PCBs and polycyclic aromatic hydrocarbons (PAHs)—charred meat is one source. Still other xenoestrogens come from combustion by-products. Xenoestrogens have the effect of functioning directly or indirectly as estrogens, thereby increasing lifetime exposure to estrogens in both men and women. Moreover, they are thought to disrupt the daily cycle of melatonin, an important nighttime hormone that appears to modify estrogen effects.

Luckily, you can neutralize these powerful compounds by adding anti-xenoestrogenic foods to your diet. These include cruciferous vegetables, garlic, onions, and soy foods. For those with a family history of breast cancer, concentrates of indole-3-carbinol, a cancer-fighting phytochemical from cruciferous vegetables, may be particularly helpful. Chapter 4 offers a guide for choosing the best foods for balancing hormones.

Sun Damage and Its Effects

Sunlight contains very high-energy ultraviolet rays called UVA and UVB. Humans have evolved with a protective skin pigment called melanin that absorbs UVA and UVB wavelengths and deactivates free radicals generated by sunlight. Consequently, darker skin that contains higher levels of melanin better protects people from sun damage. Sunrays that aren't intercepted penetrate the skin's outer epidermal layers and damage genes in the basal skin layers. These are living skin cells that are rapidly dividing and differentiating into the various types that make up the epidermis and its supporting network.

Sunbathing is a favorite occupation of young people, although damage from sun exposure usually isn't evident until years later. Yet the well-documented harmful effects of UV light exposure, whether intentional or unintentional, are a major health issue. When we're between the ages of 28 and 35, we begin to see the effects of sun exposure on our skin as wrinkles, rash, various types of lesions, and reduced elasticity. While these effects are unattractive, they don't necessarily indicate a life-threatening condition.

However, dermatologists are reporting alarming numbers of people under 20 who have developed melanoma, the most serious kind of skin cancer, which can spread to other parts of the body. The best safeguard against this is to protect the skin from infancy by reducing sun exposure, wearing protective clothing, and applying a good sunscreen. For aging skin, there are cosmeceutical remedies that will improve appearance, speed healing, and delay onset of new wrinkles and lesions.

Internal Effects of Skin Damage

The internal effects of skin damage occur through genetic damage and altered gene expression. Free radicals generated from the sun, environmental exposure, stress, and poor diet attack skin cells and cause the release of inflammatory promoters. These in turn damage your genes and increase cross-linking of collagen, making it less pliable and resilient. Free radicals change the way your cells communicate via hormones and receptors. They interfere with transport of nutrients and elimination of toxins. Dark brown age spots called lipofuscin, an accumulation of toxins, begin appearing on the skin surface, usually in areas with the most sun exposure. Bad as it is, sun damage isn't the worst thing you do to your skin every day. You should view your skin as the most important part of your body, which is in dynamic equilibrium with the rest of your body's organs. Your skin cells along with those in your internal organs integrate the nutritional and metabolic events of your life. Let's examine the impact of nutrition on your skin.

Nutrition and Your Skin

Sugar is the worst thing for your skin. Every doughnut, candy bar, and soda adds to a toxic excess of blood sugar or glucose that shows up on your face! Frequent consumption of refined carbohydrates, which are ubiquitous in the American diet, bump up cortisol levels, interfering with hormone balance and increasing inflammation (see chapter 4). Sugar also raises blood levels of insulin, the hormone that regulates sugar metabolism, and at the same time reduces sensitivity of cellular insulin receptors to glucose. Glycation or cross-linking of proteins is stepped up, collagen weakens, and wrinkles deepen. Glycation ultimately causes production of extremely toxic by-products known as advanced glycation end products (AGEs).

Sugar causes fat to accumulate in your belly, making it harder to maintain a trim appearance, particularly if you are over 40. As your waistline girth increases, so does your risk of heart attack and stroke.

When you look in the mirror, you'll see fine lines appear that deepen over time. Sugary foods and alcohol will cause the skin above and under your eyes to puff up. Puffiness is also increased if you aren't drinking enough water. You especially need to increase your intake of fresh mineral water when traveling. Many travelers also find it helpful to carry a small mister containing mineral water for frequent spraying while flying.

Amazingly, following the dietary guidelines in chapter 4, which involves increasing your intake of lean protein and foods high in omega-3, omega-6, and omega-9 oils (fish, nuts, seeds, dark green vegetables, olive, flax, and hemp oils), will reduce the lines and puffiness within just a few days! Controlling stress is also crucial in reducing skin wrinkling and puffiness. Now let's move on to the topical remedies that will change your appearance and improve your health.

Topical Makeovers

In chapter 2, we first presented the idea of using an inside/outside approach in the Anti-Aging Solution. The previous four steps in the 5-Step Plan have shown how you can enhance DNA repair, reduce inflammation, and reestablish internal homeostasis through diet, exercise, stress reduction, and supplementation.

Now we will detail the use of topical creams to deliver cosmeceuticals that prevent further damage to your skin, reduce wrinkling, and improve body shape through hormone balancing. Liposomal creams are the ideal vehicle for delivering these nutrients because they

- Allow absorption of nutrients that might not otherwise occur.
- Can be compartmentalized: water- and lipid-soluble nutrients in separate compartments all within a single liposome. Whereas hormones are lipid soluble, CAEs and other cosmeceutical agents are water soluble. For maximum utilization, water- and fat-soluble fractions should be separated.
- Contain a lipid bilayer structure just like skin cells, making them exceptionally healing and smoothing in their own right.
- Can be easily dispensed in a measured-dose pump system.

Topical Gene Repair

The health-protecting effects of oral administration of CAEs are by now quite well documented in the scientific literature, but topical applications are just beginning to be understood and appreciated. Ozone layer thinning allows more UV light to penetrate our atmosphere, causing cosmetic companies to increase their search for natural compounds that could protect us from sunlight and overcome the deleterious effects of exposure to its rays.

Happily, cutting-edge research has surfaced, namely reducing UV-induced skin damage by enhancing DNA repair. Although a popular idea, there has been scanty evidence that it could work in a commercial product—that is, until CAEs were tested on cultures of human skin exposed to UV sunlight.

The in vitro test demonstrated that CAEs enhanced DNA repair by 79.4 percent, and as a result the number of sunburned skin cells was reduced by 95.5 percent. This is indeed welcome news. Not only can you help prevent DNA damage by applying transdermal cream containing CAEs before UV exposure but you can also overcome the effects of sun exposure by enhancing DNA repair.

CAE extract is the active ingredient in a new line of skin and body care products that repair genes in the basal layers of your skin epidermis. For the first time, it is possible to reduce signs of aging on your skin and body by changing genetic expression in the deepest layers of skin cells. Epidermal cells on the surface layers are no longer living, while those in the deeper layers are rapidly growing. CAE extract's protective and healing effects target these cells. As rejuvenated cells grow toward the surface layers of your skin, you will appear more youthful. The specific effects of CAEs on basal layers of skin cells include

- Protecting DNA in skin cells from oxidative damage
- Increasing skin cell DNA repair, even after overexposure to sun
- Boosting immune protection of skin against toxins and microbes
- Reducing skin lesions (anti-tumor effects)
- Restoring healthy apoptosis
- Blocking NF-κB and TNFα, thereby reducing inflammation
- Providing protection against UV radiation
- Protecting lipid membranes in skin cells from free radical damage
- Modifying gene expression
- Normalizing hormonal communication and signal transduction
- Decreasing inflammatory prostaglandin PGE2

By reducing inflammation through several of the processes listed above, CAEs dramatically reduce skin wrinkling, reddening, rashes, and eczema. They reduce sun damage and help repair damage, sunspots, and lesions that may have occurred years earlier. By repairing DNA and altering gene expression, CAEs help protect against serious forms of skin cancer. Topical CAE is an integral part of a good photoprotective program that includes using sunscreens, wearing protective clothing, and limiting sun exposure. The beneficial effects of topical CAEs are enhanced with supplements of lipoic acid, vitamin C, particularly ascorbyl palmitate, and vitamin E complex. The role of these vitamins is fully described in chapter 6, and they are included in your core supplement program.

Photoprotection

The use of topical sunscreen preparations is the best-known photoprotective approach. When applied regularly, sunscreens help prevent penetration of UV light into skin cells, which could otherwise have disastrous health consequences. In a recent study, scientists estimated that lifetime daily use of sunscreen between April and September alone provided protection equivalent to a 40-year reduction in exposure over a 70-year life span. There are two types of UV light that can reach your skin: UVA and UVB. UVB is the more damaging of the two, and most sunscreens do a good job of absorbing it before it reaches the skin. Few sunscreens are effective against UVA. Scientists lack a simple measure of UVA's impact on the skin, making it difficult to determine how much UVA protection a sunscreen provides. Until this is resolved, be cautious in your exposure to the sun.

While sunscreens sit on the surface of your skin, CAEs, being water soluble, penetrate your skin surface and are active in deeper skin layers where UV damage is most dangerous. Before going out in sunlight, apply cream containing CAEs along with an effective sun block. Apply the cream again after sun exposure. Look for cosmeceutical products in the near future containing CAEs and other cosmeceuticals that enhance their effects.

The DNA repair effects of CAEs in topical creams are augmented by the addition of other nutrients such as zinc, lipoic acid, fat-soluble vitamin C (ascorbyl palmitate), carotenes, and niacinamide. Glycolic acid and other alpha-hydroxy acids can also protect skin. Nicolas Perricone, M.D., and colleagues in the Department of Dermatology, Yale University, investigated the photoprotective and inflammatory effects of topical glycolic acid. Dr. Perricone demonstrated that a 50 percent solution of glycolic acid applied 15 minutes before sun exposure provided a sun protection factor (SPF) of 2.4. Dr. Perricone and his team found that a 12 percent glycolic acid cream reduced reddening and irritation in sunburned skin by 16 percent. Furthermore, daily treatment with two products containing 8 percent glycolic acid protected skin from sun. Dr. Perricone has formulated skin products based on his research. You will find them listed in the resources section.

Face and Body Makeover—Inside and Outside

Making over your skin and body will give you these benefits:

- Enhance your facial muscle tone
- Reduce redness, broken capillaries, and swelling
- Repair collagen and elastin, and prevent their breakdown
- Repair sun damage
- Reduce brown age spots and skin lesions
- Heal sunburned skin

Incredibly, dietary change and oral nutraceutical supplements alone can enhance skin quality to a remarkable level. When topical nutraceutical preparations such as CAE extract and natural hormones are added that can directly enhance DNA skin repair, there is an even greater skin rejuvenation effect by combining inside and outside DNA repair enhancement.

Transdermal Liposome Delivery Systems

Skin is a natural barrier to absorption, and it's difficult to get vital nutrients to penetrate deeper skin layers. However, we recommend a transdermal cream that utilizes a unique liposome technology. A liposome is a spherical particle composed of a closed-membrane lipid bilayer similar to that in your cells. Its building blocks are molecules that have two distinct preferences for solubility. The hydrophilic part is water soluble while the hydrophobic part is oil soluble.

The liposome is well suited to function as a cosmeceutical delivery vehicle because both the hydrophobic bilayer and the enclosed water compartment can be used to solubilize active substances. Thus, both hydrophobic and hydrophilic substances can be incorporated in a liposome. In addition, this delivery system protects vital nutrients as they move to absorptive sites in deeper skin layers to invigorate new cells. This highly effective system also provides for the slow release of actives, protecting skin for extended time periods.

Liposomal Hormone Balancing

In prior chapters, you have seen that hormones play a vital role in the aging process, and three of the previous steps in the Anti-Aging Solution—stress reduction, diet, and supplements—have addressed hormones. Now let's discuss the specifics of how male and female hormones are affected by aging and how it's possible to restore hormone balance through the use of natural liposomal hormone creams.

Male Hormones and Aging

Testosterone is the predominant male hormone, with the greatest quantities secreted in the testes. Smaller amounts are also secreted in the adrenals and ovaries. Testosterone has numerous functions:

- Development of male body and sexual characteristics
- Maintenance of male libido and sexual performance

- Building and maintaining muscle mass
- Burning fat
- Maintaining optimal skin function
- Maintaining bone density and strength
- Maintaining immune function
- Promoting and sustaining mental performance

Both men and women make testosterone from two hormone precursors, the primary one being progesterone. It's interesting to note that progesterone, normally considered a female hormone, is the source for testosterone. A second precursor for testosterone is dehydroepiandrosterone (DHEA). The body makes DHEA from androstenedione (andro), a popular supplement for athletes. Testosterone is converted into other hormones, namely the three estrogens and 5-dihydrotestosterone (DHT). A balance between testosterone and estrogens is an important factor in male aging.

As men reach their mid-thirties, levels of testosterone begin declining, but estrogen levels remain about the same. This causes a relative decrease in the ratio between testosterone and estrogens (T/E), which is responsible for the changes in body composition and male personality characteristics that occur during andropause. However, this isn't the only reason for the shift in the T/E ratio. There are other reasons why this shift may intensify:

- Age-related increases in aromatase activity (the enzyme that converts testosterone into estrogens)
- Alteration in liver function (through toxin buildup)
- Zinc deficiency
- Obesity
- Overuse of alcohol (raises estrogen levels by interfering with their elimination from the body)
- Drug-induced estrogen imbalance (beta-blockers, cimetidine)
- Ingestion of estrogen-enhancing foods (beef, dairy products, fatty foods)
- Endocrine disrupters

Body and Personality Changes

Young men typically have high energy levels and assertiveness associated with a high ratio of testosterone to estrogen. By middle age, the T/E ratio is about half what it formerly was and is accompanied by lower energy and fat accumulation around the waistline (love handles) and in the chest (gynecomastia). Male sexual drive and libido may also begin to lag. Male behavior typically becomes more passive and tolerant, which is probably a good thing, since this is the time of life when many fathers are facing the challenges of teenage children and perhaps a wife going through menopause.

In older men, the T/E ratio has slipped even further, leading to increasing midline girth and breast tissue enlargement. There is a marked loss of muscle and bone. Many men also experience a lethargic state of mind and in some cases clinical depression.

Lifestyle habits, particularly high alcohol intake, increase estrogen and accelerate these aging changes. Alcohol interferes with the liver conversion of estrogen into waste products. Thus, higher levels continue to circulate in the bloodstream, causing the changes mentioned. Zinc deficiency can also contribute to changes. In zinc deficiency states, the aromatase enzyme system converts more testosterone into estrogen. Finally, as men age, more testosterone is converted into the less active DHT, which occupies receptor sites and prevents free testosterone from binding. DHT does not have the signaling capability equivalent to that of testosterone and therefore does not activate important second messengers within the cell and nucleus.

Changes in Face and Skin

Testosterone maintains thick, well-nourished skin on the face and body. Years of exposure to sun's rays begin to take their toll as leathery, dry skin starts replacing the moist, supple skin of youth. These changes are accelerated among smokers. Skin lesions begin to appear and scars heal more slowly. Inflammatory skin conditions such as seborrhea and eczema may appear. High cortisol levels contribute to wrinkling and sagging skin including that on the neck. Facial and body hair becomes finer and increasingly sparse. DHT causes hair loss and prostate problems, which are common in older men. Low testosterone levels may cause

- Increased fat accumulation around the midsection of the body and breasts
- Loss of muscle or inability to maintain muscle mass
- Fatigue and low stamina
- Low sexual drive
- Depressed mood and indecisiveness

- Hair loss
- Loss of bone mass

Transdermal Natural Hormone Replacement

Delivery of hormones using creams, gels, and patches is the most efficient way to administer them. There are several reasons for this. Hormones that are swallowed will be partly degraded by the digestive system. Therefore, an allowance for this loss must be made in determining dosage. This is imprecise because of wide variation in digestive capacity among individuals. Absorbability from the intestine into the bloodstream is another factor that's hard to control, and in older individuals, it may be significantly reduced. This results in fecal elimination of actives.

After absorption, hormones must pass through the liver, where they undergo metabolism. Some will be attached to ligands that eliminate them through urine. While many drugs rely on liver metabolism to activate them, natural hormones are already active because they are bioidentical to those your body manufactures and processes.

Transdermal delivery is more convenient than taking pills. Absorption through the skin provides a time-release mechanism for absorption directly into the bloodstream. Liposomes deliver hormones that are hydrophobic, along with augmenting hydrophilic cosmeceuticals such as CAEs through the epidermis and into the bloodstream. Finally, creams and gels offer a distinct advantage over patches in that they are not visible.

A Note on Steroid Therapy

All hormones are steroids because they're derived from cholesterol. Yet we generally think of steroids either as medications such as cortisone or for athletic enhancement. Their use is controversial, whether prescribed on not. Consequently, we want to point out two hormones we will mention, DHEA and androstenedione, because they are particularly controversial due to misuse. There are sound therapeutic reasons and research to support their use when appropriate. However, they are often used solely to enhance athletic performance, causing the International Olympic Committee (IOC), the National Football League (NFL), and the National Collegiate Athletic Association (NCAA) to all ban the use of DHEA. The IOC also bans the use of androstenedione. The following discussion is extremely important within the context of anti-aging, and the recommendations are based on your results of home test kits as presented in the appendix A.

Transdermal Progesterone

Progesterone is the basic hormone for producing androstenedione, testosterone, and estrogens. In men, progesterone reduces the conversion of testosterone into dihydrotestosterone (DHT), the latter a factor in the development of prostate cancer. Progesterone also reduces inflammation in benign prostatic hypertrophy. In appendix A you will learn about saliva testing for male hormones.

Dr. Norman Gonzales of Tampa Bay, Florida, suggests a transdermal progesterone cream (20 mg twice daily) that can be applied to the abdomen and genital area in men to help prevent prostate conditions and andropause symptoms. Younger men may only need 10 mg applied twice a day, if saliva tests show testosterone levels are not significantly lowered.

DHEA

Dehydroepiandrosterone and its sulfated form DHEA-S are produced in the adrenal cortex and converted into the active androgens (male hormones) testosterone and its immediate precursor, androstenedione. DHEA is rapidly converted into DHEA-S, and this is the primary circulating form. Both of these hormones can be subsequently converted into estrogen. The lack of DHEA-S has been closely associated with aging. Peak levels occur during the mid-twenties; thereafter, levels decrease until they are almost nonexistent by the time a man reaches his eighties.

The importance of DHEA has mostly been attributed to being a precursor of testosterone. However, a growing body of evidence suggests that an important function of DHEA is balancing cortisol levels. Both of these hormones decline progressively and markedly with aging, although aging effects on the adrenal cortex and slower clearance of cortisol from the liver keep cortisol levels from dropping as much as those of DHEA.

DHEA has a number of important effects that are important in the anti-aging plan. It is well established that it enhances immune system efficiency. It plays an important role in cancer prevention and immune response to vaccination. DHEA also increases thermogenesis and thus burning of fat. While caloric restriction has been shown to increase longevity, DHEA augments this effect, possibly through increasing the efficiency of insulin but also by reducing appetite.

DHEA enhancement of insulin function increases lean muscle mass and improves the sensitivity of cellular insulin receptors. Insulin resistance is an underlying cause of obesity and diabetes.

DHEA plays an important role in cardiovascular health by preventing platelet aggregation and generation of arterial plaque. Finally, DHEA sustains cognitive function, elevates mood, and increases your sense of well-being. Low levels of DHEA have been associated with dementia, Alzheimer's, and memory loss in men. Following is a summary of DHEA functions:

- Enhances immune function
- Balances cortisol levels
- Improves stress adaptation
- Has anti-inflammatory properties
- Reduces risk of cardiovascular disease
- Burns fat
- Increases lean muscle
- Enhances brain function
- Improves insulin receptor sensitivity and reduces risk of diabetes

Deficiencies of DHEA in men have been associated with

- Reduced immunity
- Psychological depression
- Poor memory
- Low metabolic rates and low energy
- Low estrogen levels
- Low HDL (good) cholesterol
- Increased risk of cancer
- Increased risk of cardiovascular disease

As you can see, low levels of DHEA share some of the same effects as low levels of testosterone. Consequently, the male saliva hormone test panel we suggest in appendix A includes both hormones in addition to androstenedione, estriol, and progesterone. Low levels of DHEA can be raised either with oral supplementation or transdermal delivery creams.

Transdermal DHEA

Scientists in the Department of Reproductive Medicine, University of California, San Diego, did a series of studies that included men and women ages 40 to 70. DHEA supplementation increased serum DHEA to youthful levels as well as insulin-like growth factor 1 (IGF-1), a measure of increase in growth hormone release. This was associated with a significant increase in perceived physical and psychological well-being. In another study, the UCSD researchers found that a longer period of supplementation and higher doses increased androgenic hormones including testosterone, DHT, and androstenedione.

Moreover, the lower the DHEA levels at the beginning of the study, the greater the increment of IGF-1. Men also gained physical strength as demonstrated by knee extension/flexion, increased lean muscle mass, and reduced body fat. These same effects were not observed in women.

Finally, a small group of men with an average age of 67 were given DHEA and tested for immune function by checking the activity of two groups of immune cells: T lymphocytes (T cells) and B lymphocytes (B cells). Several specialized kinds of T cells fight infection and protect tissues that have been injured. B cells produce antibodies that recognize bacteria and viruses to which they have been previously exposed. Antibodies recruit T cells and other immune complexes to attack pathogens quickly and aggressively. The activity of both groups of immune cells was dramatically enhanced without one kind being preferentially increased to the detriment of others.

Using transdermal delivery of DHEA in appropriate measured doses appears to induce anabolic growth factors, increase muscle strength and lean body mass, activate immune function, and enhance quality of life in aging.

Female Hormones and Aging

Female hormones are produced in the reproductive organs, adrenal glands, and fat tissue. During pregnancy, a significant amount of estrogen is converted from DHEA-S. Estrogen is a group of three hormones: estradiol (E_1), estriol (E_2), and estrone (E_3). Of these, estradiol is the most potent, estriol less so, and estrone the least potent. After menopause, estrone becomes the major estrogen, as the adrenal glands play a more important role in hormone production than the ovaries.

Estrogens work in balance with progesterone to support female reproduction and develop secondary sexual characteristics such as breast development and body fat distribution. The following table summarizes the balance between these two groups of hormones:

Estrogen Effects	Progesterone Effects
Endometrial proliferation	Endometrial secretions
Growth of endometrium	Maintenance of endometrium during pregnancy
Stimulates breast tissue	Protects against breast fibrocysts
Increases body fat deposition	Burns fat for energy
Causes salt and fluid retention	Natural diuretic
Increases depression and headaches	Anti-depressant action
Interferes with thyroid hormones	Enhances thyroid action
Increases blood clotting	Normalizes blood clotting
Decreases libido	Restores libido
Impairs blood sugar control	Normalizes blood sugar levels
Retention of copper, zinc loss	Restores zinc and copper balance
Reduces cellular oxidation	Restores proper oxygen levels
Increases risk of endometrial cancer	Prevents endometrial cancer
Increases risk of breast cancer	Helps prevent breast cancer
Restrains osteoclast bone resorption	Stimulates osteoblast bone building
Reduces vascular tone, increasing migraines and varicose veins	Protects myelin sheath on nerves

Source: Adapted from John Lee, M.D. *Natural Progesterone—The Multiple Roles of a Remarkable Hormone.* BBL Publications, Sebastopol, California, 1993. Reprinted with permission.

Shifts in hormone balance both before and after menopause contribute to your sense of physical, mental, and emotional well-being. Premenstrual and menopausal symptoms are commonly treated with synthetic hormone replacement.

Menopause has traditionally been viewed as estrogen deficiency, and estrogen replacement therapy (ERT) has been a common treatment. Paradoxically, progesterone drops to nearly zero after menopause while estrogens are merely diminished. In the mid-1970s, it was recognized that giving estrogen without progesterone increased the risk of cancer, particularly in women who had an intact uterus. Consequently, doctors began giving synthetic progestins along with estrogen. The most common form of prescribed estrogen is Premarin, a combination of estrogens that occur naturally in horses but are not natural in the human body.

However, because these estrogens are not bioidentical to human estrogens, they are not metabolized in the same way. Oral progesterone was first used as HRT in 1934, but the liver rapidly degraded most of it. Consequently, synthetic progestins were developed in the 1940s. However, synthetic hormones are more potent than their natural precursors and remain active in the system for extended periods. This translates into significant side effects. It has been found that the active metabolites of synthetic hormones can cause significant damage to DNA, which is one way they contribute to cancer. Another is by creating free radicals that damage DNA.

Progestins are not bioidentical to progesterone, and side effects have caused many women to abandon them. Reports of breast tenderness, weight gain, bloating, and irregular bleeding are the most common. Moreover, progestins have not been found to have the same benefits as progesterone. In one study, postmenopausal women with reduced exercise capacity due to cardiac ischemia were given natural estrogen with either progestins or progesterone. Progestins did not enhance the protective benefits of estrogen. Natural progesterone, in contrast, increased the benefits of estradiol significantly.

Doctors have used HRT to relieve symptoms of menopause based on evidence that it protects women from cardiovascular disease and bone loss. While HRT does reduce menopausal symptoms such as flushing and helps prevent osteoporosis, it does not protect against cardiovascular disease.

Alarming signs that the benefits of HRT might be outweighed by its risks were announced in July 2002. The Women's Health Initiative (WHI) involved 16,608 menopausal women, ages 50 to 79, who were enrolled in the study for 5.2 years. The women were given either Pempro, a combination of synthetic estrogens and progestins, or placebo. The study was halted 3 years early because the women who were given Pempro had more strokes, heart attacks, blood clots, and an increased risk of invasive breast cancer than those receiving the placebo. The HRT users did experience benefits including reduced bone loss and reduced incidence of colorectal cancer, but these did not outweigh the risks.

Based on the results of this and other studies that questioned the wisdom of widespread HRT use, especially for protection against cardiovascular disease, physicians were advised by medical experts such as Andrew Kaunitz, M.D., editor of *Medscape Women's Health Journal,* to use caution in recommending HRT and not use it to prevent cardiovascular disease. It was suggested that doctors should find other therapies to prevent bone loss. Additionally, they should advise their patients on benefits of dietary change, exercise, maintenance of normal weight, moderation of alcohol intake, and smoking cessation to reduce menopausal symptoms.

Physicians were further advised to recommend calcium and vitamin D supplements to prevent bone loss. Many women have been confused about what to do about menopause symptoms and their long-term health. Consequently, many have looked for natural alternatives to HRT.

Fredi Kronenberg, Ph.D., of the Rosenthal Center for Complementary and Alternative Medicine, College of Physicians and Surgeons, Columbia University, and Adriane Fugh-Berman, M.D., of the Department of Health Care Sciences, School of Medicine, George Washington University, reviewed twenty-nine randomized, controlled clinical trials of complimentary and alternative medicine or CAM therapies for hot flashes and other menopausal symptoms. The doctors found that soy foods provide modest relief for hot flashes among most women and soy isoflavones also have some benefit.

Among herbal remedies, black cohosh *(Cimicifuga racemosa)* also helped reduce menopausal symptoms, especially hot flashes. They found inconsistent results with other popular remedies including vitamin E, dong quai *(Angelica sinensis),* and evening primrose oil. Consequently, Kronenberg and Fugh-Berman suggested black cohosh and foods containing phytoestrogens were the best CAM therapies to alleviate many of the symptoms of menopause. See chapter 4 for food suggestions to alleviate menopausal symptoms and chapter 6 for helpful supplements. However, natural hormone replacement may offer the most immediate benefits.

Topical Hormone Balancing with Progesterone

Topical creams containing progesterone are well absorbed and can be useful in rebalancing hormones in both men and women. Transdermal progesterone contains the bioidentical hormone that's found in your body. It is rapidly absorbed into the bloodstream and can be easily converted into other hormones on an as-needed basis. Natural progesterone is more easily eliminated from the body once adequate levels are achieved, and this makes it safer to use than other hormone preparations.

In women, transdermal progesterone reduces the deleterious effects of excess estrogen. Progesterone increases apoptosis, thus augmenting the effects of CAEs and reducing the incidence of breast cancer. It also dramatically reduces the symptoms of perimenopause.

Perimenopause is defined as the transition between a woman's reproductive years and menopause when menstruation ceases completely. Perimenopause typically occurs between the ages of 40 and 51 and may last anywhere from 6 months to 10 years. This period is characterized by estrogen dominance with fluctuations in progesterone levels. It produces symptoms commonly encountered during perimenopause including breast tenderness, uterine fibroids, heavy or breakthrough bleeding, more frequent or irregular periods, and headaches. Although estrogen dominance is common during perimenopause, it can occur at any time in a woman's life.

According to John Lee, M.D., progesterone cream can offset the following symptoms of estrogenic syndrome:

- Early puberty
- Irregular menses
- Endometriosis
- Autoimmune conditions
- Fibromyalgia
- General fatigue
- Water retention
- Weight gain around thighs and buttocks
- Depressed mood
- Low libido

Ignacio Armas, M.D., an obstetrician/gynecologist specialist from Puerto Rico, suggests women use 20 mg of transdermal progesterone cream twice daily, increasing it to 60 mg (20 mg three times per day) if needed to control symptoms. A pump system that delivers measured doses of transdermal progesterone is highly effective and the most convenient to use.

Transdermal DHEA

Anti-aging effects of DHEA have been documented in women alone, and in those studies reviewed previously on DHEA supplementation in men. There are, however, differences between the genders in DHEA metabolism. An interesting study was done at the University of Tennessee, Department of Obstetrics and Gynecology, in which a significant increase in insulin sensitivity was found among middle-age women but not among men supplemented with DHEA for 3 weeks. Thus, DHEA may offer an important treatment for insulin resistance. It was also noted that DHEA balanced stress effects on the brain. This was confirmed in another study that demonstrated DHEA balances the deleterious effects of stress on brain function. DHEA decreases by about 60 percent in postmenopausal women. Since this hormone and to a lesser degree androstenedione are the precursors for both estrogen and androgens, increasing levels of DHEA can result in increased bone formation and higher bone mineral density. DHEA also appears to inhibit the growth of some types of breast cancer.

In addition to the hormones discussed for men and women, melatonin is important in delaying aging.

Melatonin, Your Hormonal Time Keeper

The pineal is a small endocrine gland about the size of a kernel of corn that sits above and slightly behind the hypothalamic/pituitary axis (HPA) in the center of your brain. The pineal is the first organ to be formed during the earliest weeks following conception. Originally, scientists thought the pineal was a vestigial organ, a relic of our evolutionary past, with no useful purpose. However, since the late 1970s it has been increasingly recognized that the pineal is a fundamental modulator of the entire neuroendocrine system.

The pineal gland functions as a true biologic clock secreting its hormone melatonin in a circadian fashion. The pineal gland and melatonin are capable of translating environmental lighting information into signals that modulate reproductive, adrenal, and other neuroendocrine interactions as well as immune function.

Melatonin levels rise after sunset and levels peak between 2 and 5 A.M. Levels drop rapidly once the sun rises, dropping to baseline by 8 A.M. The circadian rhythm can be disturbed by changes in temperature, humidity, light exposure, jet lag, and even magnetism. For millennia we have depended on natural light to synchronize our biological clock. The introduction of artificial light and late nighttime TV viewing or computer work may be a significant cause of altered melatonin release and sleep problems. Shift workers and those living in extreme northern climates also experience poor synchronization of biological clocks.

Moreover, the 24-hour rhythm of melatonin is very robust when we're young but declines as we age. Numerous studies now suggest that melatonin may directly or indirectly delay aging and inhibit age-related disease processes.

Stress and Melatonin

Melatonin is produced by enzymatic conversion from the amino acid tryptophan. Niacin is also produced from tryptophan, as is the calming neurotransmitter serotonin. The conversion of tryptophan into niacin isn't efficient, with 60 mg of tryptophan being utilized to produce 1 mg of niacin. Chronic stress depletes tryptophan while increasing demand for niacin to combat the stress. One reason we tend to increase carbohydrate consumption during periods of stress is that it elevates tryptophan levels, and, as a consequence, serotonin levels. Stress-induced depletion of tryptophan leads to lowered levels of melatonin and serotonin. Melatonin is nature's anti-stress hormone because it counters the effects of high cortisol. Yet continued stress induces a vicious cycle:

Increased cortisol → decreased tryptophan →
decreased serotonin → decreased melatonin →
increased cortisol → accelerated aging → aging conditions

The cycle may be reversed with therapy using melatonin and perhaps tryptophan or its metabolite 5-hydroxytryptophan (5-HTP) plus niacin and pyridoxine.

Melatonin Effects on DNA

Melatonin readily crosses all membrane barriers, and many scientists consider it to be the best antioxidant known. In one animal study, rats exposed to the carcinogen safrole sustained 41 to 99 percent less DNA damage when they were given melatonin prior to exposure. Melatonin is a powerful scavenger of oxygen free radicals. It thus prevents oxidative damage to DNA and activation of NF-κB, which in turn promotes a cascade of inflammatory mediators, as described in chapter 2.

Mitochondrial DNA is particularly susceptible to oxidative damage. We have seen that reducing caloric intake is an important anti-aging strategy because burning calories to produce energy generates harmful oxidative radicals within the mitochondria. The more calories consumed, the greater number of free radicals that will be generated as a normal by-product of metabolism. Melatonin enhances the anti-aging effects of caloric restriction because it protects mitochondrial DNA from oxidative damage.

Melatonin and Immune Function

Some years ago it was established that in humans the immune and hematopoietic (blood cell–forming) systems operate with circadian rhythms. This affects not only the number of cells produced but also their function. Receptors for melatonin were found on immune cells, suggesting the hormone activates them. It was also found that melatonin activates the second messengers within immune cells. There is evidence of a bidirectional interaction between immune cells and the pineal gland in that certain immune modulators act on the pineal.

Both melatonin and immune-protective IgA (immunoglobulin A) are elevated at night following daytime bright light exposure, suggesting nighttime is an important recovery period for the immune system. It has been found that melatonin does indeed have a direct effect on the immune system and that disturbances in melatonin release, in some cases by medications such as beta-blockers (propranolol), should be allowed for in treatment for cardiovascular conditions.

Furthermore, there is evidence that melatonin interacts with the hypothalamus by stimulating the release of thyrotropin-releasing hormone (TRH). This hormone acts upon the pituitary to release thyroid-stimulating hormone (TSH). Both of these hormones appear to prevent loss of thymus gland function, and by doing so, help preserve youthful T-cell development. Thyroid function is intimately associated with that of other endocrine glands. Low levels of thyroid hormones are common in middle-age and older individuals. It has also been suggested that alterations in female hormone cycling might be caused by low levels of melatonin. Of particular interest in aging is the occurrence of shortened menstrual cycles in perimenopause. We suggest you test your saliva melatonin levels, particularly if you have sleep problems.

Melatonin Deficit and Other Aging Conditions

Menopause is associated with a decreased secretion of melatonin and an acceleration of bone loss. There is considerable evidence that pineal gland function is linked to osteoporosis.

- Melatonin delays the aging process and certain aging conditions.
- Melatonin secretion decreases sharply during menopause.
- Melatonin opposes the osteoporotic effects of cortisol.
- Melatonin inhibits synthesis of prostaglandin E_2, which is implicated in bone loss.
- Melatonin secretion increases with exercise and decreases with immobility.
- Osteoporosis is delayed with chronic sunlight exposure. Osteoporosis is accelerated during winter months.

Consequently, scientists have suggested that testing melatonin levels during early menopause may be a useful indicator of susceptibility to osteoporosis.

Disturbances in melatonin release and cortisol have been documented in a number of aging conditions including Parkinson's, excessive sleep (hypersomnia), narcolepsy, delayed sleep syndrome, and periodic restless leg syndrome.

Transdermal Melatonin

Melatonin is lipophilic (fat-loving), allowing for rapid transdermal uptake and distribution throughout body tissues and fluids. It is ideal for coordinating physiological rhythms upset by aging, chronic stress, or immune system dysfunction. Melatonin has been used to relieve depression, seasonal affective disorder (SAD), and neurodegenerative disorders such as Parkinson's and Alzheimer's. Because it is a powerful and global antioxidant, melatonin may reduce susceptibility to aging conditions such as cancer, cardiovascular disease, and diabetes.

Stories Your Face and Body Tell

Your face and body have much to tell about DNA repair capability and hormones in aging. Following is an overview of the aging signs you see in the mirror, what they mean, and what you should order in your saliva home test kit as detailed in appendix A.

Who Is Affected	What You See	What It Means	Tests to Order
Men and women	Wrinkles	Altered ratio between collagen and elastin, protein cross-linking	Saliva panels: Stress, Men's or Women's Panel A
Women	Fine lines around eyes and lips	Estrogen deficiency	Saliva panels: Women's Panel A
Men and women	Chin "wattles," sagging jowls	Free radical damage, drop in collagen synthesis, increased damage to skin proteins, inflammation, low hormone levels	Saliva panels: Stress, Men's or Women's Panel B
Men and women	Puffiness around eyes	High cortisol, poor digestion, dehydration	Saliva panels: Anti-Aging Extreme Stress Panel
Men and women	Loss of muscle tone, excessive accumulation of body fat on trunk and extremities	Reduced insulin receptor sensitivity, increased levels of insulin and cortisol	Saliva panels: Anti-aging Stress Panel, Athlete
Men and women	Concentration of fat in abdomen; pear shape or "beer belly"; rest of body may not be fat	Syndrome X, high LDL and low HDL, increased uric acid, low insulin	Saliva panels: Men's or Women's Panel B
Men	Breast enlargement, fat in upper chest	Low levels of testosterone, growth hormone	Saliva panels: Men's Panel B
Women	Breast enlargement	Excess estrogen and progesterone, with higher ratios of progesterone to estrogen	Saliva panels: Women's Panel A
Women	Breast size decreased, sagging	Low estrogen and progesterone, loss of insulin receptor sensitivity, blood sugar elevation	Saliva panels: Women's Panel B, Stress

Prescription for Skin and Body Makeover

The information presented here may seem a little confusing in that it seems we are suggesting you may need several of these creams for your face and body makeover. The positive changes you will see in the mirror are the result of all 5 steps in the DNA repair plan. We are also suggesting that you will benefit from transdermal application of CAEs. However, use of any of the other creams discussed in this chapter will depend on the results of your saliva test. All of the following recommendations should be followed only until saliva hormone levels are restored to normal range. The transdermal creams are applied to any soft-tissue area of the body such as underarms, thighs, belly, or face and neck.

Men

Skin lesions, wrinkling, rashes: Use transdermal CAEs with augmenting nutrients such as niacin, zinc, lipoic acid, and ascorbyl palmitate. Apply daily in the morning or before and after sun exposure.

Low testosterone or low androstenedione: Use transdermal androstenedione with augmenting nutrients such as chrysin, *Tribulus terrestris,* saw palmetto extract, damiana extract, selenium, zinc, and grapeseed extract to prevent conversion of testosterone into DHT. Apply daily.

High estrogen: Use progesterone (10 mg) applied twice daily.

Low DHEA: Use DHEA cream, 15 mg twice daily, or 25 mg oral DHEA twice a day. (Oral doses are higher than topical doses because the liver converts some oral DHEA into inactive metabolites.)

Low melatonin: You may either use melatonin cream, 3 mg applied before bedtime, or take 1 to 3 mg oral or 500 mcg sublingual melatonin just until sleep is restored or saliva melatonin levels are normal.

Women

Skin lesions, wrinkling, rashes: Use transdermal CAEs with augmenting nutrients such as niacin, zinc, lipoic acid, and ascorbyl palmitate. Apply daily in the morning or before and after sun exposure.

Low estrogen, progesterone, or high testosterone: Use transdermal progesterone, 20 mg applied in the morning and again in the evening.

Low DHEA: Use DHEA cream 15 mg once daily or 25 mg oral DHEA every other day. (Oral doses are higher than topical doses because the liver converts some oral DHEA into inactive metabolites.)

Low melatonin: You may either use melatonin cream, 3 mg applied before bedtime, or take 1 to 3 mg oral or 500 mcg sublingual melatonin just until sleep is restored or saliva melatonin levels are normal.

You should consult your physician when you receive your saliva test results regarding the best course of action in your particular case. It may be advisable to have a compounding pharmacist prepare transdermal creams with natural hormones for you. For example, you must have estrogen, testosterone, and thyroid hormones prescribed for you because they are not available over the counter. If you do not have a physician who is versed in natural anti-aging medicine, you may wish to consult with one of the physicians listed in our medical consulting service, Profile Health, in the resources section.

Testing for Hormone Levels

Saliva tests give an overview of your levels of hormones and the balance that exists between them. Based on the results of your tests, you can design a program for natural hormone replacement. Unlike synthetic hormones, natural hormones and their precursors are bioidentical to those your body produces. They can be directly utilized by your cells or converted into other needed forms by your body. They are virtually nontoxic and have no side effects. The transdermal delivery system ensures rapid uptake and assimilation of the hormones into your system. The appendix explains home testing.

Conclusion

Take Charge Today!

Like many others, you may have been discouraged by not finding the medical help you sought to alleviate signs and symptoms of aging. You're not content to accept that you're just growing older and you have decided to take charge of your own aging and do whatever you can to maintain a long, healthy life.

If you already look years younger than your biological age, you may have been considering how to keep these "youth genes" going strong. Or if you look older than you'd like, perhaps its time to find out why and overcome the visible signs of aging. *The Anti-Aging Solution* provides the necessary answers to take charge of your life.

You have no doubt already become curious about the anti-aging success stories of Dr. Giampapa's patients who you have met throughout this book. Gerri's story is particularly significant.

> I came to Doctor Giampapa almost 4 years ago feeling somewhat desperate. I had gone through some really bad times and the stress was taking a toll on my body. My cholesterol was up to 284 (normal is below 200). My weight was on a steady incline and I felt out of control. I exercised faithfully and watched what I ate, so what was it I was doing wrong?
>
> Dr. Giampapa helped me take an honest look at what I was doing. Bottom line—it wasn't working. My blood serum and saliva were analyzed, and Dr. Giampapa came up with a 5-step

187

plan. Hormone imbalances were a big part of my problem, and the first thing he did was get my thyroid and insulin levels in check. Next he put me on natural topical hormone therapy because my levels were dangerously low and almost depleted. The cream included a balance of estrogen, progesterone, DHEA, and testosterone. I had always avoided taking any hormones but decided to try it for 1 year. It was surprising that a balance of several hormones was needed instead of the usual one or two. Plus, I quickly learned from Dr. Giampapa that synthetic hormones prescribed by most doctors are not the same as natural hormones and do not have side effects when taken in the proper balance. The hormones came in the form of an all-natural cream that is applied to the wrist each day—simple enough. I also used a facial cream that contained estrogen, DNA repair, and antioxidants. The next blood test showed that Dr. Giampapa was right. Everything was in balance and I felt amazing. At that point we began fine-tuning with the other 4 steps in the plan.

With a few changes to my eating habits my weight began to drop. I've gone from a size 8 to a size 2. I keep a food journal and can now figure out for myself what works for me and how food affects how I feel. I also take an anti-aging multiple formula with antioxidants. My diet is no longer about weight; it is about health. The loss of pounds is a welcome bonus.

The final step was to look at what I was doing in the gym. I thought I was doing great—at least I actually went to the gym! I would walk on the treadmill, read my book, take a class, and go out for coffee with friends. I now seriously weight train 3 days a week. I also work with a trainer to further improve my performance. My daily cardio has gone from the mundane treadmill walk to sprints and interval training. Weight training emphasis is on working small muscle groups as well as the larger ones. I am gaining balance, flexibility, quickness, and improved self-esteem with tae kwon do. Exercise is no longer a chore; it is an absolute joy. The addition of growth hormone therapy helped kick things up a notch. I am in better shape than I was in my twenties and my body is toned and fit.

Dr. Giampapa came into my life at just the right time. I was open and receptive to learn from him and determined to change my ways. Each day I spend time being grateful for the new young-looking and healthy body that I now have. I am proud of what I have accomplished and I am forever grateful to Dr. Giampapa.

You can be just like Gerri by following Dr. Giampapa's 5-Step Plan. Trapped inside your body may be a young, healthy individual struggling to surface. You too will see and feel amazing results as you solve your personal Aging Equation. You are a remarkable person with strengths and weaknesses unique to you, and you need to take an honest look at how you are living your life and what you are doing that's contributing to your aging. Don't just pick on something you're displeased with such as being overweight. Yes, a high BMI will reduce your life span, but don't try to solve your problem with weight-loss programs that only give temporary relief.

If you seriously undertake the 5 steps in this plan, you will shed extra pounds. But that's not all you'll do. You will improve your mental outlook and bring new meaning into your life. Each day will be filled with a new appreciation of the health and vitality you are enjoying. You now have the necessary tools to take charge of your health and reduce everyday complaints. Follow the 5 simple steps faithfully and check your progress with home tests. Your success story will be an inspiration to others. Let's condense the information contained in this book into an action plan.

First, complete the health questionnaire in appendix A.

Second, send for your saliva hormone test kit and select the tests you want based on your gender, age, and lifestyle.

Third, prepare your weekly menu based on your meal plan. Set up a diary to record what you eat during the week, emphasizing more protein and fewer carbohydrates, especially late in the day.

Fourth, go shopping and purchase what you plan to eat. Go to the produce section first and fill your basket with all the different colors you see. Next, go to the fish and poultry counter and purchase your choices. Then choose organic dairy products that have no hormones. Shop for beans, whole-grain products, and brown rice. Replace herbs and spices that are more than 6 months old and purchase extra-virgin olive oil and macadamia nut oil.

Fifth, plan your exercise strategy. Make a list of the workplace exercises you plan to use and purchase any exercise videos that appeal to you from the resources section. If you go to a gym, find a personal trainer whose goals for you are consistent with what we recommend. Check into Pilates, yoga, tae kwon do, and other exercise programs that fully engage your mind in the exercise process. Gerri used to read while she did her obligatory treadmill, and it hampered her progress.

Sixth, purchase your comprehensive anti-aging multiple from a natural foods store. Insist on a formula that contains the amounts and types of vitamins and minerals listed in the recommended anti-aging multiple in chapter 6.

Seventh, purchase or borrow books and tapes on relaxation and meditation. Decide when and where you will do your twice-daily meditating. Begin by simply practicing a state of mindlessness. You may be able to do this unassisted. Follow by sending messages of appreciation to your cells for recovering from previous insults you have heaped upon them with poor dietary and lifestyle choices.

You are now ready to begin a new day in the life of your genes.

The Anti-Aging Solution Series

The Anti-Aging Solution is a series of books that will specialize in various aspects of fighting aging. We will give you sensible advice and a balanced viewpoint on the newest health guidelines, and we'll keep you informed on the latest medical advances and how you can use this information to expand your personal 5-Step Plan.

Research on the activity of carboxyl alkyl esters (CAEs) and augmenting nutrients is an active area of investigation in Dr. Pero's lab at the University of Lund in Sweden. The clinical applications of this cutting-edge anti-aging medicine are ongoing at the Giampapa Institute. Dr. Giampapa is committed to training other physicians in the methods he has successfully implemented with his patients. There are a growing number of physicians who are specializing in this new medical paradigm and they come from many parts of the world. Thus, the information we have presented in this book will be reaching not only the layperson but also his or her physician.

The Future of Anti-Aging Medicine

The practice of anti-aging medicine is in its infancy. As genome research continues to reveal new information, better methods for determining your own genetic peculiarities will emerge. This is a truly exciting area of medical research and practice—one that will be rapidly changing to meet the demands of a generation of men and women willing to take charge of their own health destiny and seeking the guidance to do so.

In the very near future you will be able to swab the inside of your cheek and collect tiny DNA chips. These will be analyzed for specific genetic variations that will help factor your personal Aging Equation. Specific recommendations for how to overcome genetic expression of these variances will be given so that you can modify your 5-Step Plan.

Meanwhile, nutrition research continues to reveal the powerful ability of food components to modify disease processes, and the food industry is applying new product standards for reduction of harmful components including trans fatty acids and sugars. Menu offerings in some restaurants are heart-friendly and smaller portion sizes are becoming a new trend.

Mind/body medicine is emerging in the new frontier of brain cell regeneration and stem cell implantation. A new understanding of neuroleptic drugs is emerging. Medicines are being patterned after natural components such as resveratrol that control aging and improve cognitive function. Anti-aging physicians are increasingly recognizing natural food and herbal components, many of which are now available as dietary supplements. We will keep you informed about other promising anti-aging agents and healthy trends as they occur.

APPENDIX A
ANTI-AGING HOME TESTING

The home test kits described in this appendix will help identify important risk indicators in your personal Aging Equation. It is not absolutely essential that you order these tests. Although home test kits have been available for monitoring blood sugar levels and detecting pregnancy and allergies for years, this is the first time a consumer has been able to monitor his or her own aging and disease risk factors.

The tests are convenient to use in your own home, relatively inexpensive, available commercially, and fully validated by research laboratories. The success of anti-aging therapies can be difficult to determine because you may not always feel any better or worse. Even if you have noticed a definite improvement in the quality of your life since implementing the Anti-Aging Solution 5-Step Plan, symptoms are likely to gradually change their intensity and be quite subjective.

Hence, over time it is important to have an independent objective measure of such improvement to aid your judgement. For example, the plan is designed to be optimal for an average-size person having an average mixture of genetic and metabolic factors, so it is likely there will be a need to fine-tune your program to optimize it for your maximal health benefit.

With the home test kits you will now be able to monitor and reliably ensure your progression toward a longer, healthier life and validate the benefits of the Anti-Aging 5-Step Plan. We suggest you do the tests as you begin the program, then retest after you have been following the plan for 12 weeks. In many cases, you will note a dramatic improvement in test results in just 2 weeks.

There are three groups of tests in your home test kit:

1. The serum thiol test for DNA repair capacity and overall health
2. The F_2-isoprostane test for oxidative burden
3. The saliva hormone panels for hormonal assessment of endocrine status

There are many tests available that are used by physicians practicing complementary medicine. Some assess cellular levels of vitamins and minerals, which give a clearer picture of functional nutrition. Others check amino acid serum levels and their metabolites in urine. Still others use stool samples to check for digestive capacity and abnormalities in intestinal function. Perhaps you are already familiar with some of these. However, the tests we have chosen are the best because they are

- Sensitive indicators of your overall health and longevity
- Cost-effective
- Convenient to use
- A good way to validate the effectiveness of your DNA repair plan

The tests we are recommending strongly complement one another and provide a broad-spectrum evaluation of biological events that signal aging. They are relatively non-invasive user-friendly procedures requiring only samples of serum, saliva, or urine. Moreover, they reveal early signals of aging events that follow the pathway to disease. These signals manifest even before any disease symptoms or feelings of ill health may be noticed. The home tests establish a hierarchy for assessing your aging.

Dr. Pero developed the serum thiol test to estimate DNA repair levels, which in turn controls the DNA damage that leads to mutation, altered gene expression, and eventual disease. F_2-isoprostanes are direct indicators of oxidative burden, which marks the cause-and-effect pathway to inflammation and autoimmunity, the principal aging diseases. Hormone panels are the quantitative measure of your body's signaling and communication system, which directly modulates health or disease.

These three tests provide you with a snapshot in time by which you can judge your health condition, regardless of whether aging conditions remain dormant or you are experiencing physical signs of aging. They are an important component of the anti-aging plan because they take the guesswork out of self-evaluation. They also provide continuous encouragement to fight aging.

These tests each require an individual test kit that you can obtain from sources recommended in the resources section of this book. For the thiol test, you either have your blood drawn or prick your finger and send the kit to a commercial lab for analysis. The F_2-isoprostane test utilizes a kit of urine dipsticks that you purchase and read at home.

The saliva hormones are also collected at home and sent to the commercial lab listed in the resources section for analysis.

Serum Thiol Test: A Measure of Longevity

As you have found out in earlier chapters, DNA damage and poor DNA repair leads to genetic mutations and altered genetic expression. This is the primary cause of aging and of chronic age-related diseases. DNA damage accumulates from a number of sources:

- Occupational exposures, radiation, or sunlight
- Genetic predisposition to cancer
- Drug resistance
- Aging
- Inflammation and pro-inflammatory cytokine production
- Immune dysfunction
- Enhanced DNA damage from immune stimulation (i.e., TNFα, IL6, CRP; see chapters 1 and 2)

Free radical attack is considered the forerunner of genetic damage and initiation of pro-inflammatory processes that promote many diseases including cancer, which is totally dependent on DNA damage. Consequently, measuring your genetic repair capability is an excellent indicator for how well you are aging and what is your risk of having an active disease condition.

The thiol test also measures how well nutritional or other therapies are working to overcome an unhealthy state or condition. For example, those who are exposed to extremely high levels of toxins could monitor their serum thiols to determine how toxin exposure has resulted in DNA damage and could monitor the effectiveness of detoxification therapy as evidenced by increasing thiol levels. People who are apparently healthy might check their thiols to determine their risk for developing a disease that runs in their family, even though disease symptoms may not yet be present. Thus, the thiol test is a health risk assessment tool. It can be repeated frequently to see how your health is improving by practicing the 5 daily steps in the Anti-Aging Solution.

What Are Thiols and How Do They Work?

Biologically occurring thiols are a sensitive indicator of oxidative damage to your DNA repair enzymes. During periods of oxidative stress, the thiol bonds that are located within folds of DNA repair enzymes are oxidized (degraded), resulting in the inability to repair your genes. Thus, measuring thiol levels in your blood serum will give you a good idea of the amount of genetic damage you have sustained from oxidative and inflammatory processes that have been at work in your body.

The thiol status of serum proteins and DNA repair enzymes has been associated with longevity in many species of mammals. Two important studies have been published that show the value of the thiol test as a measure of life span and the importance of successful nutritional intervention in aging.

The first study was carried out in 17 different mammalian species including 25 humans. The main objective was to demonstrate if levels of serum thiols were correlated with life span. It was found that humans—having the longest life span of the various species examined, estimated to be 95 years—had much higher serum thiols than shorter-lived species such as mice and rats, which live about 2–3 years. This test provided an important basis for associating serum thiol levels with life span, thus confirming their use as a surrogate indicator of DNA repair capability.

The life-span data from this study have been strongly reinforced by results from patients who have had their serum thiols tested. The ultimate goal of early detection bioassays such as those in the home test kit is to determine when we are beginning to age, delay its progression, and avoid onset of disease by faithfully following the Anti-Aging Solution 5-Step Plan.

The second study was the first clinical use of the serum thiol test as a tool for evaluating patient programs in an anti-aging nutritional therapy program. It involved healthy people between the ages of 35 and 55. They were supplemented for 4 weeks with either of two formulas: a comprehensive anti-aging nutraceutical formula or the same formula with CAE extract added. Both formulas were designed by Vincent Giampapa, M.D., whose approach was to combine as many of the known antioxidant nutritional factors into one formulation as possible while avoiding nutrient interaction. The first formula used in the study provided 39 well-known bioactive ingredients that were carefully balanced to provide nutritional support while avoiding competition between nutrients. The ultimate goal was to create a broad-spectrum blend that would address nutritional deficiencies no matter what they might be. The second formula contained the same ingredients but with 350 mg of a patented water-soluble CAE extract standardized to 8 percent CAEs added. The participants did not make any dietary or lifestyle changes during the 10-week test period.

The participants in the study had blood samples analyzed for DNA damage, DNA repair capacity, and presence of inflammatory cytokines at the beginning of the study and again 4 weeks into the supplementation period. Following 2 weeks without supplements, blood samples were again collected and analyzed. The final phase of the study included another 4-week period of supplementation followed by blood analysis.

Both formulas were very effective at reducing DNA damage in the participants' white blood cells, but the results were more pronounced in those who were also supplemented with CAEs. A reversal of aging was indicated by an increase in serum thiols. This was due to a combination of reduced DNA damage by antioxidants and enhanced DNA repair. Inflammatory cytokines were also reduced in some of the participants. The remarkable finding in this study is that while a very well-designed anti-aging supplement protected DNA and spared it further damage, the addition of CAEs enhanced DNA repair capacity, making the supplement even more effective.

These two studies suggest that higher levels of serum thiols correlate with a longer expected life span and can be used to monitor individual progress while implementing the Anti-Aging Solution 5-Step Plan.

How to Collect Your Sample

You can order your test kit from the commercial laboratory listed in the resources section. The kit comes with a form to be filled out, and you should do this before going to the clinical lab in your community to have your blood drawn. Because the laboratory doing the test is a research facility, you can have your blood drawn and submit your sample without a doctor's order. The lab may charge a small fee for drawing and processing your blood.

It is best not to have eaten for at least 4 hours before the blood draw. Going before work in the morning or at lunchtime might be convenient. Ask the lab to spin your sample for ten minutes at 2,000 rpm. Package the sample in the prepared mailer and send it for next-day delivery to the lab. Schedule your blood draw Monday through Thursday so that the sample will arrive during standard business hours. Results from analysis of your test sample are usually available within 10 days.

F_2-Isoprostane Test for Oxidative Burden

F_2-isoprostanes (F_2-IsoPs) measure oxidative stress, the primary factor in aging. You have read throughout this book about the effects of oxidative damage to DNA, particularly that of the mitochondria. F_2-IsoPs will tell you if you need additional antioxidant support. The test is noninvasive and inexpensive.

L. Jackson Roberts, M.D., and Jason D. Morrow, M.D., of the Department of Medicine, Vanderbilt University, Nashville, Tennessee, discovered unique prostaglandin-like compounds in 1990 that they characterized as F_2-IsoPs. Since then, the analysis of F_2-IsoPs has been refined and is extremely reliable. The test offers these advantages over other tests for oxidative stress:

- F_2-IsoPs are specific products of fatty acid oxidation.
- They are stable, allowing for accurate detection in the urine.
- F_2-IsoPs are present in all body tissues, so normal ranges can be established.
- They increase dramatically in animals and humans subjected to oxidative stress.
- Antioxidants significantly reduce F_2-IsoPs, whereas cyclooxygenase-inhibiting drugs are ineffective.
- F_2-IsoP levels are not affected by the amount of fat in the diet.

F_2-IsoPs are formed from oxidized arachidonic acid, one of the major fatty acids in membranes. They are extremely potent and alter membrane receptor activity, which as you have read, has a profound effect upon the life of the cell.

Certain products of fatty acid oxidation known as prostaglandin E2 (PGE2) have long been recognized as promoters of oxidative stress and inflammation. Yet, F_2-IsoPs are produced in much greater numbers than pro-oxidants of the PGE2 class and thus present a greater cause of inflammatory conditions. Fortunately, F_2-IsoPs are controlled by natural antioxidant defenses in your body. However, the numbers may exceed the capacity of internal antioxidants, particularly as one ages, and may require additional antioxidant supplements, dietary modification, and stress reduction techniques—all steps in your Anti-Aging Solution.

Gladys Block, Ph.D., a well-known epidemiologist from the University of California at Berkeley, investigated the distribution and extent of oxidative damage in a random group of people. Dr. Block and her team examined dietary, demographic, and lifestyle factors in order to identify sources of oxidative burden and better understand its role in disease. About 300 healthy adults ages 19 to 78 were enrolled in the study. The participants were instructed not to take any dietary supplements or eat additional servings of fruits and vegetables for 5 weeks prior to the study. Study participants were allowed to continue smoking and drinking moderate amounts of alcohol, if this was their practice. Nonsmokers were allowed their normal contact with smokers. The researchers chose two methods of measuring oxidative damage, one of them being F_2-IsoPs.

They found that overall women had higher levels of F_2-IsoPs than men, with obesity being the second most important factor associated with high levels of F_2-IsoPs in both genders. High levels of F_2-IsoPs were also correlated with high C-reactive protein, indicating that oxidative stress and inflammation will likely occur together. Similarly, high F_2-IsoPs accompanied high cholesterol. Study participants with the highest levels of vitamins C and E had the lowest levels of F_2-IsoPs, and high fruit intake was associated with reduced oxidative burden.

One of the most interesting findings from the study was that age did not seem to be a factor in amounts of F_2-IsoPs generated. The researchers understood that while oxidative damage to DNA accumulates with age, oxidative damage to fatty acids occurs because of other factors such as obesity, inflammation, and high cholesterol. From previous chapters, you have learned that while these conditions are aging factors, they can occur in young individuals.

A research team from the Division of Clinical Biochemistry and Human Metabolism, University of Texas Southwestern Medical Center, in Dallas, Texas, tested F_2-IsoP levels in diabetic patients. Oxidative burden and fatty acid oxidation are involved in diabetes and its microvascular complications. F_2-IsoP levels were significantly elevated in diabetics, even among those who did not have microvascular complications. The researchers also found that supplementation with 1,200 IU of natural vitamin E for 3 months significantly lowered F_2-IsoPs. The scientists suggested that the urine test for F_2-IsoPs is a fast and sensitive way to monitor this condition and is more reliable than other tests currently used.

How to Collect Your Sample

F_2-IsoPs can be tested in your home using a kit of urine test strips. The test gives you immediate feedback on what certain lifestyle practices are having on your health and longevity. You will have a day-to-day measure of your oxidative burden so that you can make appropriate adjustments in your 5-Step Plan including what levels of antioxidants are most appropriate. The test is very reliable and convenient. Details on where to obtain the strips are given in the resources section.

Saliva Tests for Hormones

Saliva has many diagnostic uses, and saliva hormone testing has become increasingly accepted as convenient, noninvasive, and reliable. Since the mid-1980s, doctors have used saliva for frequent testing of hormones to determine fertility and monitor high-risk pregnancies and successful implantation from in vitro fertilization and embryo transfer. More recently, saliva has been used to diagnose perimenopausal and menopausal imbalances, and to a lesser extent, those following andropause. It has also proven useful in correlating estrogen levels with the risk for breast cancer in women.

Using your hormone test kit, you can collect your sample at home in a stress-free environment. Saliva hormone levels correlate well with serum levels of active hormones, making self-testing an easy way for you to determine your hormone levels and monitor the effects of your Anti-Aging Solution. If you have been using hormone therapy, you can test your saliva to make sure your medication is not creating imbalances. Saliva analysis is a highly sensitive test in which individual hormones can be easily separated and quantified.

Saliva hormones, unlike most hormones in serum, are not bound to proteins, so analysis determines the free and active hormones that reflect the free unbound fraction in serum. Free hormones are biologically active and available to target tissues. Saliva tests are a selective marker for active hormone status.

How to Collect Your Sample

There are six saliva test panels, and you will choose one or two based on how the description for each panel fits your particular situation. Sample collection is simple. The kit you will purchase contains very small capped tubes for collecting your saliva. Collect your sample first thing in the morning, and don't drink (water is okay), or brush and floss your teeth before collecting your sample, as these will interfere with the test. Wash and dry your hands thoroughly before handling the tubes and collecting your sample. Be especially careful that you do not have any hormone residue on your fingers from medications, patches, or creams. If you are using a hormonal product, you should discontinue its use for 10 hours before collecting your saliva sample.

In order to get the saliva flowing, imagine that you are sucking on a sour lemon. As the saliva flows, collect it in the required number of tubes for the tests you wish to order. Cap the filled tubes tightly, wipe off the outside with a damp cloth, and put the tubes in the mailing carton provided. Fill out the enclosed submittal form and send by overnight delivery to the lab. You should schedule the overnight delivery so that your sample reaches the lab and can be processed during normal business hours. This means saliva collection Monday through Thursday will be best. Your test results and normal ranges for each hormone will be sent back to you within 2 weeks. We suggest you take the results of your tests to your doctor for discussion during your next routine visit.

Men's Test Panels

As you discovered in chapter 7, an imbalance of male hormones can result in fatigue, loss of muscle mass, reduced sex drive, bone loss, and depression. Two men's panels are offered. The first is for men approaching or past andropause and the second is for men concerned about prostate problems.

Unlike menopause, andropause is not characterized by an abrupt change in hormone levels. Rather, hormone levels in men drop gradually from age 35 onward. Consequently, saliva tests provide valuable information on the health and aging risks associated with lowered hormone levels.

Men's Panel A

Panel A is for men who

- Have any of the conditions mentioned above or in detail in chapter 7
- Are any age and want to determine their hormone levels
- Are concerned about the effects of endocrine disrupters
- Are planning their anti-aging program or considering hormone replacement therapy

Saliva is a very convenient method for measuring bioactive testosterone levels in the general public. Levels of bioactive testosterone decline as men age while levels of balancing hormones increase. Consequently, it is important to measure these other hormones as well.

In men, progesterone keeps estrogen in balance, particularly as they age and the balance between testosterone and estradiol is altered.

Progesterone can also serve as an important precursor of bioactive testosterone.

The saliva test establishes whether estradiol dominates over testosterone. Estrogen dominance in men is associated with male breast cancer and prostatic conditions including prostate cancer.

DHEA is an adrenal androgen, or male hormone precursor. In andropause, DHEA becomes the most important precursor of bioactive testosterone. A decrease in DHEA indicates an increased risk of cardiovascular disease in men. DHEA may also be protective against Alzheimer's disease.

Androstenedione is a major precursor of testosterone and helps boost and maintain testosterone levels. This is important for middle-age men whose natural production of testosterone decreases as a function of the aging process.

Men's Panel B

This panel identifies hormonal imbalances associated with prostate conditions and can be used to monitor the effectiveness of treatment for these conditions. It is useful for men who are

- Experiencing difficulty urinating
- Experiencing pain with bowel movements
- Currently undergoing treatment for a prostate condition

Progesterone opposes estradiol and prevents it from dominating testosterone levels. Progesterone also activates neurotransmitters, thus increasing mental function and memory. As progesterone levels decline, diminished recall of recent events increases.

Excessive levels of estradiol have been associated with tumors in testes and adrenal glands. As the ratio of estradiol to testosterone increases, men may experience breast enlargement, weight gain, reduced assertiveness, and lagging libido.

Dihydrotestosterone (DHT) is a much more powerful androgen than testosterone. It is responsible for the formation of male genitals during fetal development and for their development during puberty. And although DHT is a better anabolic agent than testosterone, too much of it causes male pattern baldness and prostate enlargement. However, as men age, less testosterone is available for conversion to DHT. Consequently, estrogen dominance rather than increased DHT is being increasingly considered as the cause of prostate problems.

Low levels of androstenedione enhance the effects of low testosterone and contribute to symptoms associated with aging in men, namely low energy, reduced sex drive, depression, and loss of muscle mass and bone density. DHEA is the primary precursor of testosterone as men age, helping to prevent estrogen dominance.

Women's Test Panels

Hormone imbalances are a common cause of discomfort in women and girls throughout life. Women approach the end of their reproductive lives at a time when they are peaking in careers and are often most stressed. Many are part of the so-called sandwich generation with teenage children and with parents who are beginning to experience serious conditions or perhaps dying. In addition to the demands of a busy lifestyle, longtime exposure to various endocrine disrupters causes further hormone imbalance.

There are two hormone panels available for women. The first is to check hormone levels in young women and during perimenopause. The second is for postmenopausal women. Too much estrogen and too little progesterone (estrogen dominance) is common during this time, causing irregular periods, shortened cycle time, and heavy bleeding. Endocrine disrupters are a common cause of estrogen dominance. The panels we are recommending are useful for women of all ages. However, the suggested panels are particularly useful for older women.

Women's Panel A

The tests in panel A are suggested for women who

- Suffer from common symptoms of PMS or perimenopause
- Have been diagnosed with uterine fibroids or endometriosis
- Are taking birth control pills, estrogen replacement therapy (ERT), or hormone replacement therapy (HRT) to monitor levels and check for imbalances
- Wish to establish baseline values before deciding about or beginning hormone therapy
- Are considering pregnancy after age 35, or have difficulty conceiving or carrying out a successful pregnancy

Increasing PMS and related symptoms are a common occurrence in perimenopause, and lowered progesterone levels underlie most of the symptoms women in this group experience. Estradiol is produced in several body sites as already discussed. Excess estrogen is conjugated (complexed) in the liver so that it can be eliminated in urine. Circulating estrogen levels increase if the liver is significantly toxic from overuse of alcohol or other pollutants.

With the onset of menopause, estrone begins replacing estradiol as the major estrogen circulating in the body. It is a less potent form of estrogen yet contributes to estrogen dominance and unpleasant symptoms of perimenopause. Like estradiol, estrone is conjugated in the liver prior to being eliminated from the body.

Women's Panel B

Menopause is technically the cessation of menses. However, as women get closer to the end of their menstruating years, symptoms of menopause become more evident. These include hot flashes, fatigue, fuzzy thinking, insomnia, and reduced immune response. A woman experiencing these symptoms is often advised by her doctor to begin ERT, or if she has an intact uterus, HRT. One form of estrogen, estrone or E_1, continues to be secreted at a lower level after menopause, while progesterone levels plummet. When the ovaries stop releasing ova, the corpus luteum, which formerly produced progesterone, no longer functions. Consequently, low progesterone levels rather than estrogen deficiency is a more likely cause of menopausal symptoms. Panel B is a more comprehensive panel than panel A and can be used by women of all ages.

The panel is most appropriate for women who

- Are experiencing symptoms of menopause
- Are postmenopausal
- Are at risk for bone loss
- Are monitoring hormone therapy
- Are monitoring the effectiveness of their anti-aging therapy
- Have had a hysterectomy

Little progesterone is secreted after menopause, and this is considered a cause of increased risk of osteoporosis. Progesterone balances estrogen and provides protection against estrogen dominance.

Estradiol and androstenedione are the major precursors of estrone. It is important to check both estradiol and estrone when either is low. After menopause, most circulating estrogen is estrone. Since it is synthesized in fat tissue, being overweight may cause significant amounts of this bioactive form, contributing to estrogen excess with binding to estrogen receptors in breast tissue and enhancing the risk of breast cancer in those who are susceptible.

Testosterone is the intermediate step in the conversion of androstenedione to estrogen. Yet high salivary levels of testosterone can indicate androgen-sensitive tumors such as those in the ovaries. Consequently, measuring bioactive testosterone levels in women is an important screening tool for detecting such tumors. High testosterone levels cause some of the undesirable effects of menopause such as increased facial hair, acne, hair loss, and deepened voice.

A decrease in DHEA-S indicates a reduced resistance to stress and an increased risk of cardiovascular disease. DHEA-S also has anti-inflammatory activity, and low levels are implicated in autoimmune conditions such as rheumatoid arthritis. Low levels are also associated with thyroid disease, diabetes, and Alzheimer's disease. Consequently, the anti-aging panel explained below is also suggested.

Anti-Aging Stress Panel

As you saw in chapter 3, chronic stress causes high cortisol levels, and in chapter 6 you found out that cortisol has been called the aging hormone. As you discovered in chapter 7, the adrenal glands are multifunctional endocrine organs that secrete a variety of hormones. These hormones control your survival when threatened with microbial attack, injury, or any life-threatening situation. They also orchestrate tissue response to injury or infection as well as regulate blood glucose levels, protein, carbohydrate, and fat metabolism, and electrolyte balance. Your adrenal glands help you adapt to an ever-changing environment.

A comprehensive saliva test should therefore include testing for high levels of cortisol and other hormone levels. These hormones are commonly out of balance in aging conditions. Consequently, you should choose the anti-aging stress panel in addition to the appropriate men's and women's A or B panel.

The anti-aging panel is a good screening tool for those who are going through stressful changes in life, whether work or family related, physical, or emotional. The panel contains four additional tests for those who are under extreme stress and have adrenal burnout. If your lifestyle includes a high-stress job, stressful personal or professional relationships, loss of a loved one, or serious financial problems, you are at risk for adrenal burnout and perhaps serious illness. Common indicators of severe stress are extreme irritability, headaches, constant indigestion, insomnia, impotence, irregular heartbeat, diarrhea, dizziness or lightheadedness, and loss of appetite. Chronic high levels of cortisol in older men are associated with osteoporosis. The panel screens for stress response, immune competence, and altered sleep patterns.

It will benefit those who are

- Monitoring response to stress-reduction techniques (chapter 3)
- Experiencing constant fatigue, sleep disturbances, or unexplained irritability
- Experiencing frequent headaches
- Experiencing frequent indigestion: acidity, bloating, gas, or loss of appetite
- Having difficulty recovering from an illness

Choose the extreme stress options if you are

- Extremely fatigued
- Battling a chronic illness: viral, bacterial, or yeast overgrowth
- Experiencing severe food allergies
- Unable to handle stress: feel trapped, depressed, or have a negative outlook
- Unable to plan and carry out events or work productively
- Experiencing severe PMS or sexual dysfunction

The daily rhythm of cortisol release is an important determinant of adrenal gland function. It normally peaks during the early morning hours, then declines steadily until midnight. By testing morning levels, it is possible to determine if cortisol levels are too low to mount an adequate stress response. Abnormally high evening levels may indicate an unremitting cycle of adrenal activation typical of chronic stress. Salivary cortisol levels can help determine serious adrenal malfunction: either too high (Cushing's disease) or too low (Addison's disease).

The ratio between testosterone and cortisol is an important indicator of the balance between anabolic (building) and catabolic (breakdown) processes in the body. Anabolic metabolism is favored by a high testosterone to cortisol ratio. High cortisol and low testosterone is indicative of accelerated aging and is associated with diabetes, cognitive dysfunction, depression, presenile dementia, and Alzheimer's disease.

As the natural counter to stress and high cortisol levels, low DHEA-S indicates a reduced adaptive response to stress and an increased susceptibility to immune dysfunction. Aldosterone is the principal mineral corticoid secreted by the adrenal glands. (See chapter 7 for more details on adrenal hormones.) Aldosterone helps regulate blood pressure, electrolyte balance, and homeostasis. It regulates potassium and sodium metabolism, and low levels result in muscle weakness, cramping, irregularities in heart rhythm, and hypertension.

Thyroid hormones regulate carbohydrate and fat metabolism and thus body weight and energy. Bioactive thyroid hormones affect growth, energy production, libido, fertility, and reproduction, as well as mental, central nervous system, gastrointestinal, and respiratory function. Of most significance in aging, thyroid hormones regulate transcription factors in gene expression. Consequently, low or elevated levels impact the most basic cellular functions.

Approximately 93 percent of circulating thyroid hormone is thyroxin or T_4. However, most T_4 is quickly converted into triiodothyronine or T_3, which is about four times more potent but has a circulating life of only one-sixth that of T_4. Saliva, unlike serum, contains only the bioactive unbound hormones. Thus, using saliva as the diagnostic tool for thyroid function is much more efficient than using serum.

Immunoglobulin A (IgA) is the dominant antibody found in mucosal surfaces such as those in your mouth, respiratory and digestive tracts. It protects these membranes from invasion by microbial agents. Levels of IgA vary from day to day, depending on stress levels, dietary factors, mood, and exercise. IgA levels drop as you age, so it is important to assess salivary levels to determine how resistant to infection you are. By keeping stress under control, eating a good diet, and exercising, you can elevate IgA.

Melatonin is a potent antioxidant and anti-aging hormone. It protects the brain against stress-induced free radical damage. Melatonin staves off the immune decline of aging, specifically by regulating TNFα and increasing IgA, interleukin-2, and T-cell activity. Consequently, low levels are extremely costly in terms of disease resistance, mental function, and longevity. Assessing salivary levels of melatonin is an effective way to decide whether adding melatonin should be part of your anti-aging program.

Competitive Athlete Panel

This panel is designed for those who are training for competition, particularly if it has been difficult to overcome a plateau in gaining strength, muscle mass, speed, or endurance. The panel is also a useful aid in assessing the effectiveness of dietary supplements. It is important to establish baseline values for hormones before beginning a new training regimen or hormone supplementation. Periodic reassessment of hormone levels is essential to prevent overtraining and to keep tabs on your progress and help you achieve your training and competitive goals.

Consider adding this panel

- To find out why you are unable to progress in training as expected
- If you are beginning an intensive exercise program
- If you are making significant changes in your training regimen
- To measure gains in your exercise program
- To monitor your steroid levels

Low levels of cortisol cause fatigue, poor stamina, allergies, and arthritis. High levels cause muscle wasting, growth retardation, osteoporosis, and immune suppression.

Testosterone is vital to maintain a competitive drive and to develop and maintain muscles. It is essential for repair of tissues and recovery from injury. Extremely high levels of testosterone in men may increase its conversion to estrogen, particularly if androstenedione is also high, leading to breast enlargement (gynecomastia).

High levels of androstenedione in women are an important indicator of excess androgens. In both men and women athletes, low levels are a primary cause of reduced energy, reduced stamina, loss of muscle mass, and reduced sex drive. In women athletes, a low ratio of androstenedione to testosterone is associated with excess facial hair growth.

DHEA-S maintains lean muscle mass and reduces fat storage. It is an active neurosteroid that primes the hippocampal brain center to maintain mood, energy, libido, and physical performance.

Following is a table that summarizes the tests we've discussed and the hormones that are assayed in each test:

SUMMARY OF HORMONES TESTED

Hormones Tested	Men's A	Men's B	Women's A	Women's B	Anti-aging	Athlete's
Progesterone	✔	✔	✔	✔		
Testosterone	✔			✔	✔	✔
DHT		✔				
Estradiol E_1	✔	✔	✔	✔		

Hormones Tested	Men's A	Men's B	Women's A	Women's B	Anti-aging	Athlete's
Estrone E$_3$			✔	✔		
Cortisol					✔	✔
IgA				✔	✔	✔
DHEA-S	✔	✔		✔	✔	✔
Aldosterone					✔*	
Thyroid T$_3$					✔*	
Thyroid T$_4$					✔*	
Melatonin					✔*	
Androstenedione	✔	✔				✔

Note: Tests checked with an asterisk are for those with extreme stress or adrenal burnout.

You have no doubt noticed that some of the hormones appear in several of the panels. You should list the panels you want, regardless of the number of times an individual hormone is listed. All hormones listed for a particular panel must be considered to reveal deficiencies, determine imbalances, and suggest appropriate remedies. However, only one test for each hormone will be run in order to avoid duplicate testing. This way you are not paying for multiple tests of the same hormone.

Costs for the Tests

The costs listed here are current through early 2004 and subject to change. You can get updated pricing from the labs performing the tests that are given in the resources section.

- *Serum thiol test:* $65.
- *F$_2$-Isoprostane test strips:* $10.
- *Saliva hormone panels:* Each hormone in the panel costs $25. Single hormone tests are $30. The test kit for collecting and submitting your sample costs $10, but this fee is refunded at the time your sample is submitted for testing.

How Do I Use These Test Results?

Serum Thiols

Thiol levels above 120 indicate that you have less than a 5 percent chance of having an active disease. Thiol levels below 90 suggest that you may have an active disease and should seek the guidance of a physician experienced in anti-aging medicine. Tests on the third level may be used to define your condition. You should carefully implement the 5 steps in the Anti-Aging Solution and retest your thiols in 12 weeks to monitor your progress.

F_2-Isoprostanes

This test is a qualitative measure of the level of free radicals you are not able to successfully neutralize. Continued oxidative burden causes aging and leads to aging conditions. Consequently, it is extremely important to reduce free radicals. Chapter 4 details antioxidant-rich foods that you must include every day in your diet. Chapter 3 offers helpful tips on stress reduction and keeping cortisol under control. Chapter 5 discusses how vigorous exercise generates large numbers of free radicals. You can find which supplements you should increase to reduce free radicals in chapter 6.

Give yourself 4 weeks on the plan, then retest your F_2-IsoPs. Since each of us responds differently to oxidative burden, this test will give you valuable feedback on what level of antioxidants you need to keep free radicals under control.

Saliva Hormone Levels

These test results provide you with valuable information on what you need to do to establish balanced metabolism. For each hormone that is outside the normal limits, you will need to make modifications in your 5-Step Plan. Keep in mind that all 5 steps will affect hormone balance and that the topical creams are just one step in the Anti-Aging Solution. Chapter 7 gives details on which cream you may choose based on your saliva test results. We also list referrals for doctors to interpret your test results in appendix C.

Tests Requested by Your Physician

Cardiovascular Panel

The next time you visit your doctor, ask for a C-reactive protein (CRP) test, particularly if you are at risk because of smoking, hypertension, overweight, or due to a family history of heart disease. This test is becoming increasingly accepted as an important general marker of inflammation. As you read in chapter 1, it is especially important for those who are concerned about heart disease, immune or inflammatory conditions. The test is inexpensive and clinical labs are constantly updating normal values.

In January 2003, a panel of medical experts from the American Heart Association and Centers for Disease Control and Prevention established new levels for CRP. Concentrations of less than 1.0 mg/L are defined as low risk, 1.0–3.0 mg/L as average risk, and higher than 3.0 mg/L as high risk. Those who have the highest CRP levels have a two-fold greater risk of cardiovascular disease than those with the lowest levels.

Urine F_2-Isoprostanes

You may wish to verify the results you have gotten with your urine home test kit for F_2-IsoPs. If so, your doctor can instruct you to collect your urine and send it into the lab for analysis. The laboratory test accurately measures the quantity of F_2-IsoPs in your body. Healthy individuals should have between 1 and 2 nanograms of F_2-IsoPs per milliliter (ng/ml) of urine. Those who have high levels of free radicals—a likely indicator of accelerated aging—will have levels greater than 10ng/ml. As you embrace the Anti-Aging 5-Step Plan, free radical levels will begin to drop, indicating anti-aging benefits.

Gene SNP Screening Test

SNP testing procedures are currently available in commercial laboratories. This approach alone holds the future for delivering the ultimate in health care, namely personalized medical therapies. Some applications have already been identified that help patients. These include adjusting drug doses to compensate for individual differences in drug metabolism and identifying genetic predisposition to certain human conditions with the goal of dampening documented risk factors. Examples of this are familial history for lung, colon, and breast cancers.

The technology is also proving to be useful in designing anti-aging therapies that include lifestyle modifications such as those in the Anti-Aging Solution 5-Step Plan. If you have a family history of early onset of age-associated disease, then consult with your physician about the appropriateness of SNP testing in designing a personalized anti-aging solution.

The collection kit contains a cotton swab that is rubbed along the inside of your cheek. It is then sent to a lab for analysis. Test results will indicate variations in genes (SNPs) that lead to disordered enzyme function in specific metabolic pathways. Armed with this information, your anti-aging physician can then design a personalized program that upregulates these enzymes to help prevent disease.

You have no doubt read about using cheek swabs for DNA analysis to make associations between family members, and these tests examine a significant portion of the total genome. The SNP test analyzes only a few genes encoding enzymes that can most easily be regulated to alter risk of developing a disease to which you are susceptible.

Hormone Tests

Your doctor may want to order saliva tests for you or check the results you got from your own test kit. Saliva only contains hormones that are in the free state while serum contains primarily protein-bound hormones. Consequently, the normal range for serum hormones will be higher than that for saliva hormones. Parallel tests run on saliva and serum have shown that the two kinds of tests correlate well.

APPENDIX B
SUBJECTIVE QUESTIONNAIRE

Key: Rate each item by placing a circle around the appropriate number. Total your score for all parts. Rate yourself before beginning the Anti-Aging Solution and again in 30 days. Note the date you make your observations.

Part 1	Negative Change					At Start	Positive Change				
Mental Functions											
Daily enery levels	–5	–4	–3	–2	–1	0	1	2	3	4	5
Exercise tolerance	–5	–4	–3	–2	–1	0	1	2	3	4	5
Daily energy levels	–5	–4	–3	–2	–1	0	1	2	3	4	5
Exercise tolerance	–5	–4	–3	–2	–1	0	1	2	3	4	5
Sense of well-being	–5	–4	–3	–2	–1	0	1	2	3	4	5
Anxious	–5	–4	–3	–2	–1	0	1	2	3	4	5
Depressed	–5	–4	–3	–2	–1	0	1	2	3	4	5
Memory											
Recent	–5	–4	–3	–2	–1	0	1	2	3	4	5
Old	–5	–4	–3	–2	–1	0	1	2	3	4	5
Mentally focused (mental clarity)	–5	–4	–3	–2	–1	0	1	2	3	4	5
Improved recall (remembering names, etc.)	–5	–4	–3	–2	–1	0	1	2	3	4	5
Overall stress level (more/less and more relaxed)	–5	–4	–3	–2	–1	0	1	2	3	4	5
Skin											
Age spots on hands and feet	–5	–4	–3	–2	–1	0	1	2	3	4	5
Skin thicker	–5	–4	–3	–2	–1	0	1	2	3	4	5
Dry skin	–5	–4	–3	–2	–1	0	1	2	3	4	5

Part 1	Negative Change					At Start	Positive Change				
Skin *(continued)*											
Face (lines, tightness)	−5	−4	−3	−2	−1	0	1	2	3	4	5
Nail strength (splits, grooves)	−5	−4	−3	−2	−1	0	1	2	3	4	5
Nail growth	−5	−4	−3	−2	−1	0	1	2	3	4	5
Head hair growth, texture	−5	−4	−3	−2	−1	0	1	2	3	4	5
New head hair in bald spots	−5	−4	−3	−2	−1	0	1	2	3	4	5
Body hair: loss or gain	−5	−4	−3	−2	−1	0	1	2	3	4	5
Ruptured blood vessels, bruising	−5	−4	−3	−2	−1	0	1	2	3	4	5
Immune System											
Allergic reactions and symptoms (itching swollen eyes, etc.)	−5	−4	−3	−2	−1	0	1	2	3	4	5
Healing (gums, cuts, etc.— faster or slower)	−5	−4	−3	−2	−1	0	1	2	3	4	5
Colds and flu	−5	−4	−3	−2	−1	0	1	2	3	4	5

Part 2	Negative Change					At Start	Positive Change				
Digestive System	−5	−4	−3	−2	−1	0	1	2	3	4	5
Digestive problems (gas, bloating, constipation, diarrhea)	−5	−4	−3	−2	−1	0	1	2	3	4	5
Regular bowel movement	−5	−4	−3	−2	−1	0	1	2	3	4	5
Bulkier stools (sink in water/float in water)	−5	−4	−3	−2	−1	0	1	2	3	4	5
Skeletal System	−5	−4	−3	−2	−1	0	1	2	3	4	5
Bone and joint pain	−5	−4	−3	−2	−1	0	1	2	3	4	5
Flexibility	−5	−4	−3	−2	−1	0	1	2	3	4	5
Range of motion, ease of movement	−5	−4	−3	−2	−1	0	1	2	3	4	5
Joint swelling and redness	−5	−4	−3	−2	−1	0	1	2	3	4	5
Bone mineral density test	−5	−4	−3	−2	−1	0	1	2	3	4	5

	Negative Change					At Start		Positive Change			
Urinary System	−5	−4	−3	−2	−1	0	1	2	3	4	5
Continency (loss of urine control, accidents)	−5	−4	−3	−2	−1	0	1	2	3	4	5
Frequent urination	−5	−4	−3	−2	−1	0	1	2	3	4	5
Getting up at night	−5	−4	−3	−2	−1	0	1	2	3	4	5
Urgency	−5	−4	−3	−2	−1	0	1	2	3	4	5
Reduced urine flow	−5	−4	−3	−2	−1	0	1	2	3	4	5
Body Composition	−5	−4	−3	−2	−1	0	1	2	3	4	5
Weight gain	−5	−4	−3	−2	−1	0	1	2	3	4	5
Weight loss	−5	−4	−3	−2	−1	0	1	2	3	4	5
Stronger abdominal muscles	−5	−4	−3	−2	−1	0	1	2	3	4	5
Firmer thigh muscles	−5	−4	−3	−2	−1	0	1	2	3	4	5
Youthful body contour	−5	−4	−3	−2	−1	0	1	2	3	4	5
Love handles and bells disappearing	−5	−4	−3	−2	−1	0	1	2	3	4	5
More endurance when exercising	−5	−4	−3	−2	−1	0	1	2	3	4	5
More strength when exercising	−5	−4	−3	−2	−1	0	1	2	3	4	5
Upper arms (underside "wings")	−5	−4	−3	−2	−1	0	1	2	3	4	5
Abdominal fat	−5	−4	−3	−2	−1	0	1	2	3	4	5
Thigh diameter	−5	−4	−3	−2	−1	0	1	2	3	4	5
Sagging under chin	−5	−4	−3	−2	−1	0	1	2	3	4	5
Facial skin tighter	−5	−4	−3	−2	−1	0	1	2	3	4	5
Sexual Status	−5	−4	−3	−2	−1	0	1	2	3	4	5
Libido level	−5	−4	−3	−2	−1	0	1	2	3	4	5
Firmer erection (men)	−5	−4	−3	−2	−1	0	1	2	3	4	5
Frequency of sexual relations	−5	−4	−3	−2	−1	0	1	2	3	4	5
Increased sensitivity	−5	−4	−3	−2	−1	0	1	2	3	4	5
Menopausal symptoms (hot/cold flashes, headaches, etc.)	−5	−4	−3	−2	−1	0	1	2	3	4	5
Periods Regular	−5	−4	−3	−2	−1	0	1	2	3	4	5
Irregular	−5	−4	−3	−2	−1	0	1	2	3	4	5

	Negative Change					At Start	Positive Change				
Sleep Function	−5	−4	−3	−2	−1	0	1	2	3	4	5
Fall asleep faster	−5	−4	−3	−2	−1	0	1	2	3	4	5
Sleep interruption	−5	−4	−3	−2	−1	0	1	2	3	4	5
Sleep throughout night	−5	−4	−3	−2	−1	0	1	2	3	4	5
More dreaming sensation	−5	−4	−3	−2	−1	0	1	2	3	4	5
Dietary Habits	−5	−4	−3	−2	−1	0	1	2	3	4	5
Sugar or sweet cravings	−5	−4	−3	−2	−1	0	1	2	3	4	5
Appetite More hungry	−5	−4	−3	−2	−1	0	1	2	3	4	5
Less hungry	−5	−4	−3	−2	−1	0	1	2	3	4	5
Frequency of meal habits (more or less)	−5	−4	−3	−2	−1	0	1	2	3	4	5
Food cravings (more or less)	−5	−4	−3	−2	−1	0	1	2	3	4	5
Thirst	−5	−4	−3	−2	−1	0	1	2	3	4	5
Drink: more water or less	−5	−4	−3	−2	−1	0	1	2	3	4	5
Crave salt: more or less	−5	−4	−3	−2	−1	0	1	2	3	4	5
Alcohol: more or less craving	−5	−4	−3	−2	−1	0	1	2	3	4	5
Caffeinated beverages: more or less	−5	−4	−3	−2	−1	0	1	2	3	4	5
Body Temperature	−5	−4	−3	−2	−1	0	1	2	3	4	5
Feel cold: more or less	−5	−4	−3	−2	−1	0	1	2	3	4	5
Feel hot: more or less	−5	−4	−3	−2	−1	0	1	2	3	4	5
Flashes: hot or cold	−5	−4	−3	−2	−1	0	1	2	3	4	5

Nutrition Habits

These questions will highlight nutrition habits you may need to change. The best answer is in bold letters. Keep a daily eating diary as you progress through the 5-Step Plan and check to see how your dietary habits are improving:

1. Daily meals. On average, how many meals do you consume per day?

   a. 3 meals with healthy snacks (2 may be sufficient for older folks who are inactive)

b. 3 meals
c. 2 meals or less
d. no regular eating pattern

2. Eating out. On a weekly average, how many meals do you eat out?
   a. 7 meals per week
   b. 5 meals per week
   c. 3 meals per week
   d. fewer than 1 per week, or rarely

3. Consumption of grains/cereals/bread products (serving size is ½ cup, 1 slice of bread, or 4 medium crackers). What is your average daily consumption?
   a. Whole grains, beans, nuts: 6 to 11 servings per day
   b. Whole grains, beans, nuts: 6 or fewer servings per day
   c. Refined grains such as white bread/rolls/processed flour: at least 6 to 11 servings per day
   d. Refined grains such as white bread/rolls/processed flour: 6 or fewer servings per day
   e. Rarely eat grain products

4. Consumption of vegetables. On average, how many servings of vegetables do you consume per day? A serving is 1 cup raw or ½ cup cooked.
   a. At least 3 to 5 servings a day
   b. Less than 3 servings per day
   c. Rarely consume vegetables

5. Consumption of fruit. On average how many servings of fruit do you consume per day? A serving size is ½ cup cut-up fruit, ½ of a large apple or equivalent, or 6 ounces of fruit juice.
   a. At least 2 to 4 servings a day
   b. Less than 2 servings per day
   c. Hardly ever eat fruit or fruit juice

6. Consumption of dairy products. A serving size is 1 cup milk, yogurt, or cottage cheese, or 1 ounce cheese (high-fat cheese: cheddar, Swiss, blue, Roquefort, Stilton, Parmesan types and full-fat cream cheese; low-fat cheese: goat, Neufchâtel, low-fat cream cheese, string cheese, and mozzarella).
   a. At least 2 servings per day
   b. Less than 2 servings per day
   c. Hardly ever consume dairy products

7. Type of dairy products. Indicate the type of dairy products you consume. Check descriptions in #6 above.
   a.   Nonfat selections only
   b.   Both low-fat and nonfat, about the same
   c.   Low-fat only
   d.   High-fat selections
   e.   Only cultured, fermented, or soured types (e.g., yogurt, kefir, cottage cheese, cheese)

8. What is your daily consumption of meats and meat products?
   a.   Consume more than 6 ounces of red meat per day
   b.   Consume less than 6 ounces of red meat per day
   c.   Consume 6 ounces or less of fish or poultry per day
   d.   Do not consume meat or meat products

9. What is your daily consumption of fats, dressings, and spreads? A serving size is 1 teaspoon of high-fat selections or 2 tablespoons of low-fat items. High-fat items are butter, margarine, mayonnaise, creamy dressings, and oils. Low-fat items are oil-and-vinegar–type salad dressings and nut butters.
   a.   Use high-fat selections (more than 3 per day)
   b.   Use high-fat selections sparingly (less than 3 per day)
   c.   Use both high-fat and low-fat about equal (less than 3 per day)
   d.   Use low-fat selections frequently (3 or more per day)
   e.   Use low-fat selections sparingly (less than 3 servings per day)

10. Convenience and snack food consumption. On average how many times per day do you eat convenience foods or fast-food items?
    a.   Never
    b.   Less than 1 time per day
    c.   More than 1 time per day

11. Use of seasonings. How do you usually season your food?
    a.   Salt, soy sauce, and spice blends
    b.   Pepper and salt-free items
    c.   Mostly spices and herbs, including pepper
    d.   Ketchup, chili sauce, and salsa

12. Consumption of water. How often on average do you drink water? A serving size is 8 ounces. Do not add in beverages such as coffee, tea, or soda.

   a.   At least 8 glasses per day
   b.   About 4 to 8 glasses per day
   c.   Less than 4 glasses per day
   d.   Seldom consume water

13. Consumption of alcohol. How often do you consume alcohol?
   a.   Never drink
   b.   2 days or less per week
   c.   3 days per week
   d.   4 or more days per week

14. Number of alcoholic beverages. On the days you drink, how many drinks do you consume? Serving size is $1\frac{1}{2}$ ounces of spirits, one 12-ounce can of beer, or 6 ounces of wine.
   a.   Never drink
   b.   1 to 2 drinks
   c.   3 to 4 drinks
   d.   More than 5 drinks

15. Caffeine. How often do you consume caffeine in your diet including coffee, tea, cola, or chocolate? A serving is 8 ounces.
   a.   Never
   b.   Occasionally, but not every day
   c.   1 to 3 servings daily
   d.   3 to 5 servings daily
   e.   More than 5 servings daily

16. Smoking status. Indicate which of the following best represents your current status.
   a.   Have never smoked
   b.   Quit smoking less than 5 years ago
   c.   Quit smoking more than 5 years ago
   d.   Smoke pipe or cigar
   e.   Smoke less than 1 pack of cigarettes per day
   f.   Smoke more than 1 pack of cigarettes per day

17. Smokeless tobacco. Do you use smokeless tobacco?
   a.   Yes
   b.   No

ANTI-AGING SOLUTION SELF-REPORT FORM

Lifestyle Parameters:	Poor Health	Good Health	Your Score; Implementing the Plan				
			Start	6 mo.	12 mo.	18 mo.	24 mo.
Smoking (packs/day)	>1	<0.1	___	___	___	___	___
Stress (meditation min/day)	0	>20	___	___	___	___	___
Exercise (hr/day) (including work-related)	0	1	___	___	___	___	___
Environment							
Sunlight (% skin protect)	0	>90	___	___	___	___	___
Toxins (% avoidance)	0	>90	___	___	___	___	___
Food							
Portions (servings)	2	1	___	___	___	___	___
Calories	>3000	<2200	___	___	___	___	___
Processed (% of diet)	>50	<10	___	___	___	___	___
Colors (% of diet)							
White carbos	>50	<10	___	___	___	___	___
Red/yellow/green fruit and veggies		>70	___	___	___	___	___
Tan carbos		10–15	___	___	___	___	___
White proteins	>40	15–20	___	___	___	___	___
Self-Assessment							
Body mass index	>35	<20–25	___	___	___	___	___
Biochemical markers							
Saliva hormones Normal range	out of range	in range	___	___	___	___	___
Urine F_2-isoprostanes Normal range	>10 ng/ml	<1–2 ng/ml	___	___	___	___	___
Serum thiols (nm/l)	<90	>120	___	___	___	___	___
Supplement choices (need to correlate with end of chapter 6)							
Antioxidants	0	+ (dose)	___	___	___	___	___
DNA repair	0	+ (dose)	___	___	___	___	___
Immune function	0	+ (dose)	___	___	___	___	___
Inflammation	0	+ (dose)	___	___	___	___	___
Gene expression	0	+ (dose)	___	___	___	___	___
Anti-aging multiple	0	+ (dose)	___	___	___	___	___
Subjective health questionnaire (Total points)			___	___	___	___	___

Your Action Plan:

Each start value < 20% of good health value = Initiate 5-Step Plan

Each subsequent value ± 20% start value = Continue 5-Step Plan

APPENDIX C
RESOURCES

Anti-aging Products

DIETARY SUPPLEMENTS
CAE—Single Ingredient
Activar AC-11
Optigenex
750 Lexington Avenue
20th Floor
New York, NY 10022
(888) optignx (678-4469)

CAE—CampaMed
Better Natural Foods Stores
ProThera
4133 Mohr Avenue, Suite 1
Pleasanton, CA 94566
(925) 484-5636
(888) 488-2488

CAE—Anti-aging Formulas
Activar Age Manager
Optigenex
(888) optignx (678-4469)

Age Manager Professional
Formerly Optigene F1, Optigene
  Professional
Optigenex
(888) optignx (678-4469)

Skin Care Products

ACTIVAR
Anti-Aging and Skin Repair
Optigenex
750 Lexington Avenue
20th Floor
New York, NY 10022
(866) optignx (678-4469)

TRANSDERMAL HORMONE
CREAMS
Life-Flo Health Products
11202 North 24th Avenue
Phoenix, AZ 85029
(888) 999-7440

Natural health food stores

AllVia Integrative Pharmaceuticals
  For Physicians
11202 North 24th Avenue
Phoenix, AZ 85029
(877) 995-8715

ANTI-AGING SKIN CARE
(888) 823-7837
Department stores including Sephora,
Nordstrom's, Henri Bendel, Clyde's on
Madison, and selected Saks and
Neiman Marcus
N. V. Perricone, M.D., Cosmeceuticals,
  Ltd.

Home Test Kits

SERUM THIOL TEST
Art Banne, Lab Director
Biomedical Diagnostic Research, LLC
8140 Mayfield Road
Chesterland, OH 44026
(440) 729-6080

F_2-ISOPROSTANE TEST STRIPS
Eric Kuhrts
Lipoprotein Diagnostics, Inc.
1109 Tannery Creek Road
P.O. Box 16
Bodega Bay, CA 94922
(707) 876-9222

SALIVA HORMONE TESTS
Anti-Aging Hormone Profile Kit
Life-Flo Health Care Products
11202 North 24th Avenue
Phoenix, AZ 85029-4745
(888) 999 7440

SALIVA TEST INTERPRETATION
Profile Health, Medical Consultations
Debra Lassiter, R.N., L.N.P.
Phoenix, AZ
(480) 488-2007

Tests for Your Doctor

SERUM PROTEIN THIOL TEST
Art Banne, Lab Director
Biomedical Diagnostic Research, LLC
8140 Mayfield Road
Chesterland, OH 44026
(440) 729-6080

F_2-ISOPROSTANES URINE OR
SERUM IMMUNOASSAY
Oxford Biomedical Research, Inc.
P.O. Box 522
Oxford, MI 48371
(248) 628-5104
800 692-4633

SALIVA HORMONE ASSAY
Hormone View Personal Hormone
   Profile
Ewald Pretner, M.D., Medical Director
AllVia Diagnostic Laboratories, LLC
11202 North 24th Avenue
Phoenix, AZ 85029-4745
(602) 864-8626

AGING ASSESSMENT (IMMUNE,
BONE, METABOLIC,
CARDIOVASCULAR)
Immunosciences Lab
Aristo Vojdani, Ph.D., Founder
   and Director
8693 Wilshire Boulevard, Suite 200
Beverly Hills, CA 90211
(310) 657-1077

Spectra Cell Laboratories, Inc.
(specialize in cell micronutrient
   analysis)
7051 Portwest Drive, Suite 100
Houston, TX 77024-8026
(800) 227-5227

Great Smokies Diagnostic Laboratory
18A Regent Park Boulevard
Asheville, NC 28806
(704) 253-0621

COMPOUNDING PHARMACIES
(REQUIRE PRESCRIPTION)
Profile Health, Medical Consultations

Debra Lassiter, R.N., L.N.P.
Phoenix, AZ
(480) 488-2007

Women's International Pharmacy
Natural Hormone Therapy
2 Marsh Court
Madison, WI 53718
(800) 279-5708
12012 N. 111th Avenue
Youngtown, AZ 85363
(800) 279-5708

Hopewell Pharmacy
1 West Broad Street
Hopewell, NJ 08525
(800) 792-6670

Locating an Anti-Aging Physician

MEDICAL REFERRALS
American Academy of Anti-Aging
   Medicine (A4M)
401 North Michigan Avenue
Chicago, IL 60611-4267
(312) 321-6869

American College of Advancement
   in Medicine (ACAM)
23121 Verdugo Drive
Laguna Hills, CA 92653
(714) 583-7666
Fax: (714) 4555-9679

Aging Research and Educational Organizations

Administration on Aging
Department of Health and Human
   Services
330 Independence Avenue, SW,
   Suite 4760
Washington, DC 20201
(202) 619-0724
Fax: (202) 619-3759

Alliance for Aging Research
2021 K Street, NW, Suite 305

Washington, DC 20006
(202) 293-2856
Fax: (202) 785-8574

Division on Aging
Harvard Medical School
643 Huntington Avenue
Boston, MA 02115
(617) 432-1840
Fax: (617) 73-4432

American Aging Association
2129 Providence Avenue
Chester, PA 19013
(610) 874-7550
Fax: (610) 876-7715

International Academy of Alternative
  Health and Medicine
218 Avenue B
Redondo Beach, CA 90277

(310) 540-0564
Fax: (310) 540-0564

International Federation on Aging
601 E Street, NW
Washington, DC 20049
(202) 434-2427
Fax: (202) 434-6458

National Council on Aging
409 Third Street, SW, Suite 200
Washington, DC 20024
(800) 424-9046
Fax: (202) 479-0735

New York Academy of Sciences
2 East 63rd Street
New York, NY 10021
(212) 838-0230
Fax: (212) 888-2894

Books

Reverse Aging Through the Miracle of Natural DNA Repair, by Ronald Pero,
   Ph.D., and Marcia Zimmerman, C.N., Nutrition Solution Press, June 2002
*Eat Your Colors—Maximize Your Health by Eating the Right Foods for Your
   Body Type,* by Marcia Zimmerman, C.N., Henry Holt, Owl Books, New
   York, 2002
The A.D.D. Nutrition Solution—A Drug-Free 30-Day Plan, by Marcia Zim-
   merman, C.N., Henry Holt, Owl Books, New York, 1999
Basic Principles: Anti-Aging Medicine and Age Management, by Vincent
   Giampapa, Giampapa Institute, Montclair, New Jersey (available from
   Giampapa Institute)
Textbook of Complementary and Alternative Medicine, by Chun-Su Yuan and
   Eric J. Bieber, CRC Press, Boca Raton, FL, 2003
Secrets of Pilates, by Sally Searle and Cathy Meeus, DK Publishing, New York,
   2001
Pilates Over 50, by Lesley Ackland Thorsons, Hammersmith, London, 2001
90-Day Fitness Plan, by Matt Roberts, DK Publishing, New York, 2001
Gentle Yoga, by Lorna Bell, Celestial Arts, Berkeley, CA, 2000
Tai Chi, by Master Lam Kam Cheum, Gaia Books, London, England, 1994
Stretching, by Simon Frost, Sterling Publishing, New York, 2002
Yoga for Wimps, by Miriam Austin, Sterling Publishing, New York, 2000
The New Yoga for People Over 50, by Suza Francina, Health Communications,
   Deerfield Park, FL, 1997
Discover Fitness, by Ross Feldman, www.discoverfitness.com

Born a Healer, by Chunyi Lin, Spring Forest Qigong, Minneapolis, MN,
www.mnwelldir.org/docs/qigong/qigong3.htm
Yoga Basics, by Mara Carrico, Henry Holt, New York, 1997
Molecules of Emotion, by Candace B. Pert, Touchstone, New York, 1997
Deep Healing, by Emmett Miller, Hay House, Carlsbad, CA, 1997
Beyond the Obvious, by Christine Page, Daniel Company, Limited, Essex,
United Kingdom, 1998
The Spiritual Universe—One Physicist's Vision of Spirit, Soul, Matter, and Self,
by Fred Alan Wolf, Moment Point Press, Portsmouth, NH, 1996

Journals

*Townsend Letter for Doctors and
Patients*
911 Tyler Street
Port Townsend, WA 98368
(360) 385-0699

Journal of Anti-Aging Medicine
Mary Ann Liebert, Inc., Publishers
2 Madison Avenue
Larchmont, NY 10538
(914) 834-3689

Newsletters

*Harvard Health Letter and Harvard
Women's Health Watch*
10 Shattuck Street, Suite 612
Boston, MA 02115

Focus on Healthy Aging
Mt. Sinai School of Medicine
Box 420235
Palm Coast, FL 32142-0235
800 829-9406

*Tufts University Health & Nutrition
Letter*
10 High Street, Suite 706
Boston, MA 02110

Environmental Nutrition
52 Riverside Drive
New York, NY 10024-6599

The Nutrition Reporter
P.O. Box 30246
Tucson, AZ 85751-0246

Nutrition News
Free to customers of nutritional stores
throughout the United States
Riverside, CA

Taste for Life
Free to customers of nutrition markets
throughout the United States
Peterborough, NH

Videotapes

Windsor Pilates
www.windsorpilates.com
(800) 618-1400

*Spring Forest Qi Gong, Spring Forest
Qi Gong Products*
www.learningstrategies.com/Qigong/
home.html
Learning Strategies Corporation
2000 Plymouth Road
Minnetonka, MN 55305
(800) 735-8273

REFERENCES

CHAPTER 1: FACTORING YOUR PERSONAL AGING EQUATION

Anderson JL; et al.; Plasma homocysteine predicts mortality independently of traditional risk factors and C-reactive protein in patients with angiographically defined coronary artery disease. *Circulation* 2000;102:1227–1232.

Black P; Berman AS; Stress and inflammation. In NP Plotnikoff, ed., *Cytokines, Stress, and Immunity.* Boca Raton, FL: CRC Press, pp 118–119.

Caruso C; et al.; Cytokine production pathway in the elderly. *Immunol Res* 1996;15:84–90.

Clark JA; Peterson TC; Cytokine production and aging: overproduction of IL-8 in elderly males in response to lipopolysaccharide. *Mechanisms of Aging and Development* 1994;77:127–138.

Cunningham MW; et al.; A study of anti-group A streptococcal monoclonal antibodies cross-reactive with myosin. *J Immunol* 1986;136:293–298.

Doria G; Frasca D; Genes, immunity and senesence: looking for a link. *Immunol Rev* 1997;160:159–170.

Gloemenkamp DG; et al.; Novel risk factors for peripheral arterial disease in young women. *Am J Med* 2002;113:462–467.

Golbasi A; et al.; Increased levels of high sensitive C-reactive protein in patients with chronic rheumatic valve disease: evidence of ongoing inflammation. *Eur J Heart Fail* 2002;4:593–595.

Jaffer FA; O'Donnell CJ; et al.; Age and sex distribution of subclinical aortic atherosclerosis: a magnetic resonance imaging examination of the Framingham Heart Study. *Arterioscler Thromb Vasc Biol* 2002;22:849–854.

Kiechl S; et al.; Chronic infections and the risk of carotid atherosclerosis: prospective results from a large population study. *Circulation* 2001;103:1064–1070.

Kiechl S; et al.; Active and passive smoking, chronic infections, and the risk of carotid atherosclerosis: prospective results from the Bruneck Study. *Stroke* 2002;33:2170–2176.

Levinson W; Jawetz E; *Medical Microbiology and Immunology,* 4th ed. Stamford, CT: Appleton & Lange, 1996, pp 106; 135–138; 187–191.

Maes M; et al.; Immune and clinical correlates of psychological stress–induced production of interferon-γ and interleukin-10 in humans. In NP Plotnikoff, ed., *Cytokines, Stress, and Immunity.* Boca Raton, FL: CRC Press, pp 40–41.

Maier SF; et al.; Psychoneuroimmunology: the interface between behavior, brain, and immunity. *Am Psychologist* 1994;49:1004–1017.

Muhlestein JB; Chronic infection and coronary artery disease. *Med Clin North Am* 2000;84:123–148.

Muhlestein JF; et al.; Cytomegalovirus seropositivity and C-reactive protein have independent and combined predictive values for mortality in patients with angiographically demonstrated coronary artery disease. *Circulation* 2000;102:1917–1923.

Ridker, PM; et al.; Inflammation, aspirin, and the risk of cardiovascular disease in apparently healthy men. *N Engl J Med* 1997;336:973–979.

Ridker PM; et al.; Comparison of C-reactive protein and low-density lipoprotein cholesterol levels in the prediction of first cardiovascular events. *N Engl J Med* 2002;347:1557–1565.

Sävykoski; née Huittinen T; Chlamydia pneumoniae infection, inflammation and heart shock protein 60 immunity in asthma and coronary heart disease. Doctoral dissertation. Dept. Med. Microb., University of Oulu, Finland. 2003.

Vojdani A; A look at infectious agents as a possible causative factor in cardiovascular disease. LabMed March–May 2003; 34: 7–11, 5–9, 24–31.

Wang TJ; et al.; Association of C-reactive protein with carotid atherosclerosis in men and women: the Framingham Heart Study. *Arterioscler Thromb Vasc Biol* 2002;22:1662–1667.

Zebrack JS; Anderson JL; Role of inflammation in cardiovascular disease: how to use C-reactive protein in clinical practice. *Prog Cardiovasc Nurs* 2002;17:174–185.

CHAPTER 2: HOW AGING OCCURS

Alberts B; Bray D; Lewis J; Raff M; Roberts K; Watson, J; *DNA Repair in Molecular Biology of the Cell,* 3rd ed. New York: Garland Publ., 1994, pp 242–251.

Alberts B; et al.; Basic genetic mechanisms. In *Molecular Biology of the Cell.* New York: Garland Publ., 1994, pp 223–242.

Ame JC; et al.; PARP-2, a novel mammalian DNA damage–dependent poly(ADP-ribose) polymerase. *J Biol Chem* 1999;274:17860–17868.

Ames B; The free radical theory of aging matures. *Physiol Rev* 1998;78(2): 547–581.

Ames B; Oxidants, antioxidants and the degenerative diseases of aging. *Proc Nat Acad Sci USA* 2003;90:7915–7922.

Ames BN; et al.; High-dose vitamin therapy stimulates variant enzymes with decreased coenzyme binding affinity (increased Km): relevance to genetic disease and polymorphisms. *Am J Clin Nutr* 2002;75:616–658.

Aravind L; et al.; Apoptotic molecular machinery: vastly increased complexity in vertebrates revealed by genome comparisons. *Science* 2001;291; 1279–1284.

Atkinson HG, ed.; Human genome decoded—Now what? *Health News—New England Journal of Medicine* 2001;7(4):5.

Balducci L; Extermann M; Cancer and aging: an evolving panorama. *Hematol Oncol Clin North Am* 2001;14(1):1–16.

Barinaga M; Life-death balance within the cell. *Science* 1996;274:724.

Barnes PJ; Adcock IM; NF-κB: a pivotal role in asthma and a new target for therapy. *Trends Pharmacol Sci* 1997;18:46–50.

Barnes PJ; Karin M; Nuclear factor-κB—a pivotal transcription factor in chronic inflammatory diseases. *New Engl J Med* 1997;336:1066–1071.

Baylin SF; et al.; Alterations in DNA methylation: a fundamental focus on healthy healing aspect of neoplasia. In *Advances in Cancer Research.* San Diego, CA: Academic Press, 1998, pp 141–196.

Beg AA; Baltimore D; An essential role for NF-κB in preventing TNFα induced cell death. *Science* 1996;274:782–784.

Bohr V; Oxidative DNA damage processing and changes with aging. *Toxicol Lett* 1998;102–103:47–52.

Boulares AH; et al.; Role of poly(ADP-ribose) polymerase (PARP) cleavage in apoptosis. Caspase 3–resistant PARP mutant increases rates of apoptosis in transfected cells. *J Biol Chem* 1999; 274:22932–22940.

Carnes B; Hayflick L; Olshansky SJ; Essay: No truth to the fountain of youth. *Scientific American,* June 2002.

Commoner B; Unraveling the DNA myth. *Harper's Magazine,* Feb 2, 2002.

Cross CE; et al.; Oxygen radicals and human disease. *Ann Intern Med* 1987;107:526–545.

Doria G; Frasca D; Genes, Immunity, and senescence: looking for a link. *Immunological Reviews* 1997;160:159–170.

Eisenberg D; Complementary and Integrative Medical Therapies: Current Status and Future Trends. Division for Research and Education in Complementary and Integrative Medical Therapies, Harvard Medical School, April 12–14, 2002.

Ershler WB, Longo DL; The biology of aging: the current research agenda. *Cancer* 1997;80(7):1284–1293.

Fernandez-Pol JA; Douglas MC; Molecular interactions of cancer and age. *Cancer in the Elderly* 2000;14(1):25–43.

Fletcher RH, Fairfield KM; Vitamins for chronic disease prevention in adults: clinical applications. *JAMA* 2002;287(23):3127–3129.

Hammarstrom P; Kelly JW; et al.; Prevention of transthyretin amyloid disease by changing protein misfolding energetics. *Science* 2003;299:713–716.

Harmon D; Aging: phenomena and theories. *Ann NY Acad Sci* 1998;854:1–7.

Herceg Z; Wang ZQ; Functions of poly(ADP-ribose) polymerase (PARP) in DNA repair, genomic integrity and cell death. *Mut Res* 2001;477:107–110.

Human Genome Project; *Science* 2001;291(5507):1177–1304.

Jimenez-Sanchez G; Childs B; Valle D; Human disease genes. *Nature* 2001;409: 853–855.

Jump DB; Dietary polyunsaturated fatty acids and regulation of gene transcription. *Curr Opin Lipidol* 2002;13:155–164.

Jump DB; Clark SD; Regulation of gene expression by dietary fat. *Annu Rev Nutr* 1999;19:63–90.

King GL, Brownlee M; The cellular and molecular mechanisms of diabetic complications. *Endocrinol Metab Clin North Am* 1996;25(2):255–270.

Kinkead G; *The Very Radical Business of Long Life and Eternal Youth.* Worth Publ., 2001, pp 1–7.

Klatz R; Anti-aging medicine: resounding, independent support for expansion of an innovative medical specialty. WorldHealth.net, 2002.

Kovacs E; et al.; Impaired DNA repair synthesis in lymphocytes of breast cancer patients. *Eur J Cancer Clin Oncol* 1986;22:863–869.

Leipzig RM, ed.; Anti-aging medicine: beyond the hype. *Focus on Healthy Healing.* Mount Sinai School of Medicine Newsletter, Nov. 2002;5:1–6.

Michaud DS; et al.; Dietary sugar, glycemic load, and pancreatic cancer in a prospective study. *J Natl Cancer Inst* 2002;94(17):1293–1300.

New Report on the Maturing U.S. Supplement Industry: Challenges Ahead for an Industry in Transition. *Nutrition Business Journal,* Sept. 30, 2002.

Packer L; Coleman C; *The Antioxidant Miracle.* New York: John Wiley & Sons, 2000, p 219.

Perillo NL; et al.; In vitro cellular aging in T-lymphocyte cultures: analysis of DNA content and cell size. *Exp Cell Res* 1993;207(100)131–135.

Pero RW; Hypochlorous acid/N-chloramines are naturally produced DNA repair inhibitors. *Carcinogenesis* 1996;17:13–18.

Pero RW; Giampapa V; Oxidative stress and its effects on immunity and-apoptosis—DNA repair as a primary molecular target for antiaging therapies, 2002 (presentation paper, unpublished).

Pero R; Zimmerman M; DNA, the origin of life. In *Reverse Aging Through the Miracle of Natural DNA Repair.* Chico, CA: Nutrition Solution Press, 2002, pp 27–34.

Pero RW; et al.; Reduced capacity for DNA repair synthesis in patients with or genetically predisposed to colorectal cancer. *J Nutr Cancer Inst* 1983;70:867–875.

Pero RW; et al.; DNA repair synthesis in individuals with and without a familial history of cancer. *Carcinogenesis* 1989;10:693–697.

Pero RW; et al.; Progress in identifying clinical relevance of inhibition, stimulation and measurements of poly ADP-ribosylation. *Biochimie* 1995;77:385–393.

Pero RW; et al.; Serum thiols as a surrogate estimate of DNA repair correlates to mammalian life span. *J Anti-Aging Med* 2000;3:241–249.

A Profile of Older Americans: 2001; Administration on Aging, U.S. Department of Health and Human Services.

Rattan SJ; Synthesis, modifications, and turnover of proteins during aging. *Exp Gerontol* 1996;31(1–2):33–47.

Reaney P; Kidney cancer growing fastest in British women. *Reuters Medical News,* Oct. 2002.

Results from the 1994–1996 Continuing Survey of Food Intakes by Individuals. Food Surveys Research Group, Beltsville Human Nutrition Research Center, Agricultural Research Service, U.S. Department of Agriculture, December 1997.

Roberts LJ; Morrow JD; Measurement of F_2-isoprostanes as an index of oxidative stress in vivo. *Free Radical Biol Med* 2000;28:505–513.

Sandoval M; et al.; Cat's claw inhibits TNFα production and scavenges free radicals: role in cytoprotection. *Free Radical Biol Med* 2000;29:71–78.

Sandoval-Chancon; et al.; Antiinflammatory actions of cat's claw: the role of NF-κB. *Ailment Pharmacol Ther* 1998;12:1279–1289.

Santos AP: The architecture of interphase chromosomes and gene positioning are altered by changes in DNA methylation and histone acetylation. *J Cell Sci* 2002;115:4597–4605.

Serhan CN; et al.; Novel functional sets of lipid-derived mediators with anti-inflammatory actions generated from omega-3 fatty acids via cyclooxygenases 2-nonsteroidal anti-inflammatory drugs and transcellular processing. *J Exp Med* 2000;192:1197–1204.

Sheng Y; et al.; Induction of apoptosis and inhibition of proliferation in human tumor cells treated with extracts of *Uncaria tomentosa. Anticancer Res* 1998;18:3363–3368.

Sheng Y; et al.; Enhanced DNA repair, immune function and reduced toxicity of C-Med-100, a novel aqueous extract from *Uncaria tomentosa. J Ethnopharmacol* 2000;69:115–126.

Sternberg M; et al.; Effects of glycation process on the macromolecular structure of the glomerular basement membranes and on the glomerular functions in aging and diabetes mellitus. *CR Seances Soc Biol Fil* 1995;189(6):967–985.

Temelkova-Kurktschiev T; et al.; Subclinical inflammation is strongly related to insulin resistance but not to impaired insulin secretion in a high-risk population for diabetes. *Metabolism* 2002;51(6):743–749.

Thomas PS; Heywood G; Effects of inhaled tumor necrosis factor alpha in subjects with mild asthma. *Thorax* 2002;57:774–778.

Travis J; The true sweet science. *Science News* 2002;161(15):232–233.

Van Antwerp DJ; et al.; Suppression of TNFα induced apoptosis by NF-κB. *Science* 1996;274:787–789.

Wang CY; et al.; TNFα and cancer therapy–induced apoptosis: potentiation by inhibition of NF-κB. *Science* 1996;274:724–727.

Warner HR; Apoptosis: a two-edged sword in aging. *Anti-Cancer Res* 1999;19:2837–2842.

Watson RE; Goodman JI; Epigenetics and DNA methylation come of age in toxicology. *Toxicol Sci* 2002;67:11–16.

Wong IH; Lo YM; New markers for cancer detection. *Curr Oncol Rep* 2002;4:471–477.

Wood RD; et al.; Human DNA repair genes. *Science* 2001;291:1284–1289.

Young VM; et al.; Effect of linoleic acid on endothelial cell inflammatory mediators. *Metabolism* 1998;47:566–572.

Zochbauer-Muller S; et al.; Aberrant DNA methylation in lung cancer; biological and clinical applications. *Oncologist* 2002;5:451–457.

CHAPTER 3: STEP 1: REDUCE YOUR STRESS

Astin AW; An integral approach to medicine. *Altern Ther Health Med* 2002; 8:70–75.

Bale TL; Giordano FJ; Vale WW; A new role for corticotropin-releasing factor-2. Suppression of vascularization. *Trends Cardiovasc Med* 2003;13:68–71.

Carrasco GA; Van de Kar LD; Neuroendocrine pharmacology of stress. *Eur J Pharmacol* 2003;463:235–272

Esch T; et al.; Stress in cardiovascular disease. *Med Sci Monit* 2002;8: RA93–RA101.

Farrar WL; Kilian PL; et al.; Visualization and characterization of interleukin-1 receptors in the brain. *J Immunol* 1987;139:459–463.

Ganong WF; The adrenal medulla and adrenal cortex. In *Medical Physiology*. Norwalk, CT: Appleton & Lange, 1993, pp 334–335, 339–340.

Greaves G; Reflections on a new medical cosmology. *J Med Ethics* 2002;28: 81–85.

Jacobs GD; The physiology of mind-body interactions: the stress response and the relaxation response *J Altern Complement Med* 2002;8:219.

Kivimaki M; Leino-Arjas P; et al.; Work stress and risk of cardiovascular mortality: prospective cohort study of industrial employees. *Brit Med J* 2002;325:1386.

McVay MR; Medicine and spirituality: a simple path to restore compassion in medicine. *Nutr Clin Care* 2002;5:182–190.

Miller, EE; Taking responsibility for your own health. In *Deep Healing—The Essence of Mind/Body Medicine*. Carlsbad, CA: Hay House, Inc. 1996, pp 55–56, 106, 137–140.

Najib T; et al.; A prospective study of sleep duration and coronary heart disease in women. *Arch Intern Med* 2003; 163:205–209.

Pert CB; *Molecules of Emotion—The Science Behind Mind-Body Medicine.* New York: Simon & Schuster, 1999, pp 269–271.

Pert CB; The wisdom of the receptors: neuropeptides, the emotions, and body-mind—1986. *Adv Mind Body Med* 2002;18:30–35.

Pert CB; Dreher HE; Ruff MR; The psychosomatic network: foundations of mind-body medicine. *Altern Ther Health Med* 1998;4:30–41.

Pokharna H; Meditation. In Yuan CS, ed., *Textbook of Complementary and Alternative Medicine.* Boca Raton, FL: Parthenon Publ. Group, 2003, pp 81–90.

Sacerdote P; Ruff MR; Pert CB; Cholecystokinin and the immune system: receptor-mediated chemotaxis of human and rat monocytes. *Peptides* 1988;suppl 1:29–34.

Salford LG; Brun AE; et al.; Nerve cell damage in mammalian brain after exposure to microwaves from GSM mobile phones. *Environ Health Perspect,* Jan. 29, 2003. http://dx.doi.org/.

Scheufele PM; Effects of progressive relaxation and classical music on measurements of attention, relaxation and stress responses. *J Behav Med* 2000; 23:207–228.

Shermer M; Demon-haunted brain. *Scientific American,* Mar. 2003, p. 47.

Simon H, ed.; Stress. CBShealthwatch.medscape.com. Sept 1999.

Stipanuk, MH; Protein synthesis and degradation. In *Biochemical and Physiological Aspects of Human Nutrition.* Philadelphia, PA: WB Saunders Co., 2000, pp 225–229.

Zouboulis CC; et al.; Corticotropin-releasing hormone: an autocrine hormone that promotes lipogenesis in human sebocytes. *Proc Natl Acad Sci USA* 2002;99:7148–7153.

CHAPTER 4: STEP 2: NOURISH YOUR GENES

Abbasi F; et al.; Relationship between obesity, insulin resistance, and coronary heart disease. *J Am Coll Cardiol* 2002;40:937–943.

Agren JJ; et al.; Fish diet, fish oil and docosahexaenoic acid rich oil lower fasting and postprandial plasma lipid levels. *Eur J Clin Nutr* 1996;50:765–771.

Ai M; et al.; Relationship between plasma insulin concentration and plasma remnant lipoprotein response to an oral fat load in patients with type 2 diabetes. *J Am Coll Cardiol* 2001;38:1628–1632.

Albert CM; et al.; Blood levels of long-chain fatty acids and the risk of sudden death. *N Engl J Med* 2002;346:1102–1103.

Anderson KJ; et al.; Walnut polyphenolics inhibit in vitro human plasma and LDL oxidation. *J Nutr* 2001;131:2837–2842.

Baum JA; et al.; Long-term intake of soy protein improves blood lipid profiles and increases mononuclear cell low-density-lipoprotein receptor messenger RNA in hypercholesterolemic, postmenopausal women. *Am J Clin Nutr* 1998;68:545–551.

Beecher GR; Phytonutrients' role in metabolism: effects on resistance to degenerative processes. *Nutrition Reviews* 1999;57:S3–S6.

Berrino F; et al.; Reducing bioavailable sex hormones through a comprehensive change in diet: the diet and androgens (DIANA) randomized trial 2001. *Cancer Epidemiol Biomarkers Prev* 2001;10:25–33.

Bianchi L; et al.; Carotenoids reduce the chromosomal damage induced by bleomycin in human cultured lymphocytes. *Anticancer Res* 1993;13: 1007–1010.

Bonnesen C; Eggleston IM; Hayes JD; Dietary indoles and isothiocyanates that are generated from cruciferous vegetables can both stimulate apoptosis and confer protection against DNA damage in humon colon cell lines. *Cancer Res* 2001;61:6120–6130.

Bravo, L; Polyphenols: chemistry, dietary sources, metabolism and nutritional significance. *Nutrition Reviews* 1998;56:317–333.

Chandra RK; Nutrition and immunology: from the clinic to cellular biology and back again. *Proc Nutr Soc* 1999;58(3):681–683.

Chandra RK; Nutrition and the immune system from birth to old age. *Eur J Clin Nutr* 2002;56 (suppl):S73–76.

Constantinou A; et al.; The dietary anticancer agent ellagic acid is a potent inhibitor of DNA topoisomerases. *In Vitro Nutr Cancer* 1995;25:121–130.

Dragland S; et al.; Several culinary and medicinal herbs are important sources of dietary antioxidants. *J Nutr* 2003;133:1286–1290.

Druckmann R; Rohr UD; IGF-1 in gynaecology and obstetrics: update 2002. *Maturitas* 2002;41(suppl 1):S65–83.

DuPont MS; et al.; Effect of variety, processing, and storage on the flavonoid glycoside content and composition of lettuce and endive. *J Agric Food Chem* 2000;48:3957–3964.

Elias MF; et al.: Lower cognitive function in the presence of obesity and hypertension: the Framingham Heart Study. *Int J Obes Relat Metab Diord* 2002; 27:260–268.

Enhancement of natural immune function by dietary consumption of Bifidobacterium. *Eur J Clin Nutr* 2000;54(3):263–267.

Erlund I; et al.; Consumption of black currants, lingonberries and bilberries increases serum quercetin concentrations. *Eur J Clin Nutr* 2003;57:37–42.

Facchini FS; et al.; Hyperinsulinemia: the missing link among oxidative stress and age-related diseases? *Free Radic Biol Med* 2000;29:1302–1306.

Facchini FS; et al.; Insulin resistance as a predictor of age-related diseases. *J Clin Endocrinol Metab* 2001;86:3574–3578.

Fahey JW; Zhang Y; Talaly P; Broccoli sprouts: an exceptionally rich source of inducers of enzymes that protect against chemical carcinogens. *Proc Natl Acad Sci USA* 1997;94:10367–10372.

Ferrara LA; et al.; Olive oil and reduced need for antihypertensive medications. *Arch Intern Med* 2000;160:837–842.

Ford ES; Giles WH; Serum vitamins, carotenoids, and angina pectoris: findings from the National Health and Nutrition Examination Survey III. *Ann Epidemiol* 2000;10:106–116.

Fraser GE; Nut consumption, lipids, and risk of coronary event. *Clin Cardiol* 1999;22(suppl 7):III 11–5.

Geleijnse JM, et al.; Inverse association of tea and flavonoid intakes with incident myocardial infarction: the Rotterdam Study. *Am J Clin Nutr* 2002; 75:880–886.

Giovannucci E; Insulin, insulin-like growth factors and colon cancer: a review of the evidence. *J Nutr* 2001;131:3109S–3120S.

Giovannucci E; Modifiable risk factors for colon cancer. *Gastroenterol Clin North Am* 2002;31:925–943.

Giovannucci E; Diet, body weight, and colorectal cancer: a summary of the epidemiologic evidence. *J Womens Health* 2003;12:173–182.

Haffner SM; et al.; Decreased testosterone and dehydroepiandrosterone sulfate concentrations are associated with increased insulin and glucose concentrations in nondiabetic men. *Metabolism* 1994;43:599–603.

Hakkinen SH; et al.; Content of the flavonols quercetin, myricetin, and kaempferol in 25 edible berries. *J Agric Food Chem* 1999;47:2274–2279.

Han DH; et al.; Relationship between estrogen receptor–binding and estrogenic activities of environmental estrogens and suppression by flavonoids. *Biosci Biotechnol* 2002; 66:1479–87.

Hu FB, et al.; Fish and omega-3 fatty acid intake and risk of coronary heart disease in women. *JAMA* 2002;287(14):1815–1821.

Jacobs DR; et al.: Fiber from whole grams, but not refined grains, is inversely associated with all-cause mortality in older women: the Iowa women's health study. *J Am Coll Nutr* 2000;10(suppl 3):3265–3305.

Jakubowicz DJ; et al.; Disparate effects of weight reduction by diet on serum dehydroepiandrosterone-sulfate levels in obese men and women. *J Clin Endocrinol Metab* 1995;80:3373–3376.

Jenkinson, A McE; et al.; The effect of increased intakes of polyunsaturated fatty acids and vitamin E on DNA damage in human lymphocytes. *FASEB* J 1999;13:2138–2142.

Jensen ME; Donly K; Wefel JS; Assessment of the effect of selected snack foods on the remineralization/demineralization of enamel and dentin. *J Contemp Dent Pract* 2000;1:1–17.

Jeong HJ; et al.; Inhibition of aromatase activity by flavonoids. *Arch Pharm Res* 1999;22:309–312.

Kaaks R; Plasma insulin, IGF-1 and breast cancer. *Gynecol Obstet Fertil* 2001;29:185–191.

Kamath AF; et al.; Antigens in tea-beverage prime human $V\gamma2V\delta2T$ cells *in vitro* and *in vivo* for memory and nonmemory antibacterial cytokine responses. *Proc Nat Acad Sci USA* 2003;100:6009–6014.

Kern Pap et al.; The expression of tumor necrosis factor in human adipose tissue. Regulation by obesity, weight loss, and relationship to lipoprotein lipase. *J Clin Invest* 1995;95:2111–2119.

Khachik F; et al.; Distribution of carotenoids in fruits and vegetables as a criterion for the selection of appropriate chemopreventive agents. In *Food Factors for Cancer Prevention*. Tokyo, Japan: Springer-Verlag, 1997, pp 204–208.

Knekt P; et al.; Flavonoid intake and risk of chronic diseases. *Am J Clin Nutr* 2002;76:560–568.

Kontiokari T; et al.; Dietary factors protecting women from urinary tract infection. *Am J Clin Nutr* 2003;77:600–604.

Kris-Etherton PM; Keen CL; Evidence that the antioxidant flavonoids in tea and cocoa are beneficial for cardiovascular health. *Curr Opin Lipidol* 2002;13:41–49.

Kris-Etherton PM; et al.; Nuts and their bioactive constituents: effects on serum lipids and other factors that affect disease risk. *Am J Clin Nutr* 1999; 70(suppl 3):504S–511S.

Lachance P; Dietary intake of carotenes and the carotene gap. *Clin Nutr* 1988;7:118–122.

Lissin LW; Cooke JP; Phytoestrogens and cardiovascular risk. *J Am Coll Cardiol* 2003;35:1403–1410.

Liu S; et al.; Whole grain consumption and risk of ischemic stroke in women. *JAMA* 2000;284:1534–1540.

Lucas EA; et al.; Flaxseed improves lipid profile without altering biomarkers of bone metabolism in postmenopausal women. *J Clin Endocrinol Metab* 2002;87:1527–1532.

Manjer J; et al.; Risk of breast cancer in relation to anthropometry, blood pressure, blood lipids and glucose metabolism: a prospective study within the Malmo Preventive Project. *Eur J Cancer* Prev 2001;10:33–42.

Marmonier C; et al.; Snacks consumed in a nonhungry state have poor satiating efficiency: influence of snack composition on substrate utilization and hunger. *Am J Clin Nutr* 2002;76:518–528.

Martin KR; Wu D; Meydani M; The effect of carotenoids on the expression of cell surface adhesion molecules and binding of monocytes to human aortic endothelial cells. *Atherosclerosis* 1999;150:265–274.

Michaud DS; Giovannucci E; Fruit and vegetable intake and incidence of bladder cancer in a male prospective cohort. *J Natl Cancer Inst* 1999;91:605–614.

Michaud DS; et al.; Physical activity, obesity, height, and the risk of pancreatic cancer. *JAMA* 2001;286:967–968.

Michaud DS; et al.; Dietary sugar, glycemic load, and pancreatic cancer risk in a prospective study. *J Natl Cancer Inst* 2002;94:1293–1300.

Middleton E; Biological properties of plant flavonoids: an overview. *Internl J Pharmacognosy* 1996;34:344–348.

Miller HE; et al.; Antioxidant content of whole grain breakfast cereals, fruits vegetables. *J Am Coll Nutr* 2000;19(suppl 3):3125–3195.

Moghadasian MH; Frolich JJ; Effects of dietary phytosterols on cholesterol metabolsim and atherosclerosis: clinical and experimental evidence. *Am J Med* 1999;107:588–594.

Muti P; et al.: Markers of insulin resistance and sex steroid hormone activity in relation to breast cancer risk; a prospective analysis of abdominal adiposity, sebum production, and hirsutism. *Cancer Causes Control* 2000;11:721–730.

Nielson, FH; Ultratrace minderals. In Shils ME, Olson JA, Shike M, eds., *Modern Nutrition in Health and Disease,* 8th ed. Philadelphia: Lea & Febinger, 1994, pp 281–282.

New SA; et al.; Dietary influences on bone mass and bone metabolism: further evidence of a positive link between fruit and vegetable consumption and bone health? *Am J Clin Nutr* 2000;71:142–151.

Noda Y; et al.; Antioxidant activity of nasunin, and anthocyanin in eggplant. *Res Commun Mol Pathol Pharmacol* 1998;102:175–187.

O'Byrne DJ; et al.; Comparison of the antioxidant effects of concord grape juice flavonoids alpha-tocopherol on markers of oxidative stress in healthy adults. *Am J Clin Nutr* 2002;76:1367–1374.

Peeters, A; et al.; Obesity in adulthood and its consequences for life expectancy: a life-table analysis. *Ann Intern Med* 2003;138:24–32.

Pelucchi C; et al.; Fiber intake and laryngeal cancer risk. *Ann Oncol* 2003;14:162–167.

Querfeld U; et al.; Effects of cytokines on the production of lipoprotein lipase in cultured human macorphages. *J Lipid Res* 1990;31:1379–1396.

Raynor HA; et al.; A cost-analysis of adopting a healthful diet in a family-based obesity treatment program. *J Am Diet Assoc* 2002;102:645–656.

Reaven GM; Insulin resistance: a chicken that has come to roost. *Ann NY Acad Sci* 1999;892:45–57.

Reaven GM; Diet and syndrome X. *Curr Atheroscler Rep* 2000;2:503–507.

Reed J; Cranberry flavonoids, atherosclerosis and cardiovascular health. *Crit Rev Food Sci Nutri* 2002;42:301–316.

Rimm AA; Hartz AJ; Fischer ME; A weight shape index for assessing risk of disease in 44,820 women. *J Clin Epidemiol* 1988;41:459–465.

Rimm EB; Ascherio A; Giovannucci E; et al.; Vegetable, fruit and cereal fiber intake and risk of coronary heart disease among men. *JAMA* 1996;275:447–451.

Rolls BJ; Morris EL; Roe LS; Portion size of food affects energy intake in normal-weight and overweight men and women. *Am J Clin Nutr* 2002;76:1207–1213.

Rosenberg Zand RS; et al.; Flavonoids can block PSA production by breast and prostate cancer cell lines. *Clin Chim Acta* 2002;317:17–26.

Saghizadeh M; et al.; The expression of TNF alpha by human muscle. Relationship to insulin resistance. *J Clin Invest* 1996;97:1111–1116.

Sang S; et al.; Antioxidative phenolic compounds isolated from almond skins *(Prunus amygdalus Batsch)*. *J Agric Food Chem* 2002;50:2459–2463.

Schlosser E; *Fast Food Nation*. New York, NY: Harper Collins Publishers, 2002.

Sellneyer, DE; et al.; A high ratio of dietary animal to vegetable protein increases the rate of bone loss and the risk of fracture in postmenopausal women. *Am J Clin Nutr* 2001;73:118–122.

Slattery ML; et al.; Trans-fatty acids and colon cancer. *Nutr Cancer* 2001;39: 170–175.

Slavin J; Jacobs D; Marquart L; Whole-grain consumption and chronic disease: protective mechanisms. *Nutr Cancer* 1997;27:14–21.

Soler M; et al.; Fiber intake and the risk of oral, pharyngeal and esophageal cancer. *Int J Cancer* 2001;91:283–287.

Solfrizzi V; et al.; High monounsaturated fatty acids intake protects against age-related cognitive decline. *Neurology* 1999;52:1563–1569.

Stoll BA; Adisposity as a risk determinant for postmenopausal breast cancer. *Int J Obes Relat Metab Disord* 2000;24:527–533.

Stoll BA; Upper abdominal obesity, insulin resistance and breast cancer. *Int J Obes Relat Metab Disord* 2002;26:747–753.

Stoner, GD; Mukhtar H; Polyphenols as cancer chemopreventive agents. *J Cellular Biochem* suppl. 1995;22:169–180.

Tang AM; et al.; Low serum vitamin B12 concentrations are associated with faster human immunodeficiency virus type 1 (HIV-1) disease progression. *J Nutr* 1997;127(2):345–351.

Teixeira SR; Potter SM; et al.; Effects of feeding 4 levels of soy protein for 3 and 6 wk on blood lipids and apolipoproteins in moderately hypercholesterolemic men. *Am J Clin Nutr* 2000;72:1588–1589.

Thornalley PJ; Isothiocyanates: mechanism of cancer chemopreventive action. *Anticancer Drugs* 2002;13:331–338.

Tulp OL; DeBolt SP; Animal model: metabolic and thermic responses to diet and environment (4 degrees C) in obesity during aging in the LA/Ntul//-cp rat. *Nestle Nutr Workshop Ser Clin Perform Programme* 1999;1:149–155.

Yang G; et al.; Population-based, case-control study of blood C-peptide level and breast cancer risk. *Cancer Epidemiol Biomarkers Prev* 2001;10: 1207–1211.

Zhang Li-Xin; Cooney RV; Bertram JS; Carotenoids enhance gap junctional communication and inhibit lipid peroxidation in C3H/10T1/2 cells: relationship to their cancer chemopreventive action. *Carcinogenesis* 1991;12:2109–2114.

Zimmerman M; *Eat Your Colors! Maximize Your Health by Eating the Right Foods for Your Body Type*. New York: Henry Holt, 2001, pp 39–125.

CHAPTER 5: STEP 3: EXERCISE YOUR GENES

Ahmed C; Hilton W; Pituch K; Relations of strength training to body image among a sample of female university students. *J Strength Cond Res* 2002;16:645–648.

Berger BG; Owen DR; Mood alteration with swimming—swimmers really do "feel better." *Psychosom Med* 1983;45:425–433.

Boreham CA; Wallace WF; Nevill A; Training effects of accumulated daily stair-climbing exercise in previously sedentary young women. *Prev Med* 2000;30:277–281.

Byrne HK; Wilmore JH; The effects of a 20-week exercise training program on resting metabolic rate in previously sedentary, moderately obese women. *Int J Sport Nutr Exerc Metab* 2001;11:15–31.

Churchill JD; et al.; Exercise, experience and the aging brain. *Neurbiol Aging* 2002;23:941–955.

Dash M; Telles S; Yoga training and motor speed based on a finger tapping task. *Indian J Physiol Pharmacol* 1999;43:458–462.

Dash M; Telles S; Improvement in hand grip strength in normal volunteers and rheumatoid arthritis patients following yoga training. *Indian J Physiol Pharmacol* 2001;45:355–360.

Dunstan DW; et al.; High-intensity resistance training improves glycemic control in older patients with type 2 diabetes. *Diabetes Care* 2002;25:1729–1736.

Focht BC; et al.; The unique and transient impact of acute exercise on pain perception in older, overweight, or obese adults with knee osteoarthritis. *Ann Behav Med* 2002;24:201–210.

Giampapa VC; Exercise and Aging. In *The Basic Principles and Practice of Anti-Aging Medicine and Age Management.* Newark, NJ: 2003, Giampapa Institute for Anti-Aging Medicine, 107–123.

Glessing DL; et al.; The physiologic effects of eight weeks of aerobic dance with and without hand-held weights. *Am J Sports Med* 1987;15:508–510.

Hansen CJ; Stevens LC; Coast JR; Exercise duration and mood state: how much to feel better? *Health Psychol* 2001;20:267–275.

Hunter GR; et al.; Resistance training and intra-abdominal adipose tissue in older men and women. *Med Sci Sports Exerc* 2002;34:1023–1028.

Ivy JL; Role of exercise training in the prevention and treatment of insulin resistance and non-independent diabetes mellitus. *Sports Med* 1997;24:321–336.

Kraemer WJ; et al.; American College of Sports Medicine position stand. Progression models in resistance training for healthy adults. *Med Sci Sports Exerc* 2002;34:364–380.

Kraus WE; et al.; Effects of the amount and intensity of exercise on plasma lipoproteins. *N Engl J Med* 2002;347:1483–1492.

Laaksonen DE; et al.; Low levels of leisure-time physical activity and cardiorespiratory fitness predict development of the metabolic syndrome. *Diabetes Care* 2002;25:1612–1618.

Leipzig RM, ed.; Free and flexible. *Focus on Healthy Aging* 2002;5:4–5.

Madanmohan; et al.; Effect of yoga training on reaction time, respiratory endurance and muscle strength. *Indian J Physiol Pharmacol* 1993;37:350–352.

Malhotra V; et al.; Effect of yoga asanas on nerve conduction in type 2 diabetes. *Indian J Physiol Pharmacol* 2002;46:298–306.

Manjunath NK; Telles S; Factors influencing changes in tweezer dexterity scores following yoga training. *Indian J Physiol Pharmacol* 1999;43:225–229.

Manson JE; et al.; Walking compared with vigorous exercise for the prevention of cardiovascular events in women. *N Engl J Med* 2002;347:716–725.

Matthews CE; et al.; Moderate to vigorous physical activity and risk of upper-respiratory tract infection. *Med Sci Sports Exerc* 2002;34:1242–1248.

McCaffrey R; Fowler NL; Qigong practice: a pathway to health and healing. *Holist Nurs Pract* 2002;17:110–116.

Messier SP; et al.; Declines in strength and balance in older adults with chronic knee pain: a 30-month longitudinal, observational study. *Arthritis Rheum* 2002;47:141–148.

Nathan PA; et al.; Effects of an aerobic exercise program on median nerve conduction and symptoms associated with carpal tunnel syndrome. *J Occup Environ Med* 2001;43:840–843.

Perri MG; et al.; Effects of group- versus home-based exercise in the treatment of obesity. *J Consult Clin Psychol* 1997;65:278–285.

Petrie D; Matthews LS; Howard WH; Prescribing exercise for your patients. *Md Med J* 1996;45:632–637.

Qin L; et al.; Regular tai chi chuan exercise may retard bone loss in postmenopausal women: a case-control study. *Arch Phys Med Rehabil* 2002;83: 1355–1359.

Rafferty AP; et al.; Physical activity patterns among walkers and compliance with public health recommendations. *Med Sci Sports Exerc* 2002;34:1255–1261.

Raghuraj P; Telles S; Muscle power, dexterity, skill, and visual perception in community home girls trained in yoga or sports and in regular school girls. *Indian J Physiol Pharmacol* 1997;41:409–415.

Robb-Nicholson C, ed.; Rotator-cuff tendonitis. *Harvard Women's Health Watch* 2002;IX:7–8.

Roth SM; et al.; Muscle size responses to strength training in young and older men and women. *J Am Geriatr Soc* 2001;49:1428–1433.

Sancier KM; Electrodermal measurements for monitoring the effects of a qigong workshop. *J Altern Complement Med* 2002;9:235–241.

Siegman AW; et al.; Anger, and plasma lipid lipoprotein, and glucose levels in healthy women: the mediating role of physical fitness. *J Behav Med* 2002; 25:1–16.

Sinaki M; et al.; Stronger back muscles reduce the incidence of vertebral fractures: a prospective 10 year follow-up of postmenopausal women. *Bone* 2002;30:836–841.

Springen K; Concentrating on the body's "core." *Newsweek;* Jan. 20, 2003.

Takeshima N; et al.; Water-based exercise improves health-related aspects of fitness in older women. *Med Sci Sports Exerc* 2002;34:544–551.

Tanasescu J; et al.; Exercise type and intensity in relation to coronary heart disease in men. *JAMA* 2002;288:1994–2000.

Tsang HW; et al.; The effect of qigong on general and psychosocial health of elderly with chronic physical illnesses: a randomized clinical trial. *Int J Geriatr Psychiatry* 2003;18:441–449.

Turner LW; Bass MA; Brown B; Influence of yard work and weight training on bone mineral density among older U.S. women. *J Women Aging* 2002;14: 139–148.

Vera-Garcia FJ; Grenier SG; McGill SM; Abdominal muscle response during curl-ups on both stable and labile surfaces. *Phys Ther* 2000;80:564–569.

Vincent KR; Braith RW; Resistance exercise and bone turnover in elderly men and women. *Med Sci Sports Exerc* 2002;34:17–23.

Vyas R; Dikshit N; Effect of mediation on respiratory system, cardiovascular system and lipid profile. *Indian J Physiol Pharmacol* 2002;46:487–491.

Wang JS; Lan C; Wong MK; Tai chi chuan training to enhance microcirculatory function in healthy elderly men. *Arch Phys Med Rehabil* 2001;82:1176–1180.

Warner SE; Shaw JM; Salsky GP; Bone mineral density of competitive male mountain and road cyclists. *Bone* 2002;30:281–286.

Westcott WL; et al.; Effects of regular and slow speed resistance training on muscle strength. *J Sports Med Phys Fitness* 2001;41:154–158.

Wirhed R; Review of relevant muscles. In *Athletic Ability and the Anatomy of Motion.* Frome, England: Wolfe Medical Publications, Ltd., 1991, pp 222–233.

Yuan CS; Bieber EJ; Alternative sports medicine. In *Textbook of Complementary and Alternative Medicine.* Boca Raton, FL: CRC Press, 2003, pp 179–196.

Chapter 6: Step 4: Supplement Your Genes

Abbati C; et al.; Nootropic therapy of cerebral aging. *Adv Therapy* 1991;8: 268–275.

Abraham GE; Flechas JD; Management of fibromyalgia; rationale for the use of magnesium and malic acid. *J Nutr Med* 1992;3:49–59.

Agren JJ; et al.; Fish diet, fish oil and docosahexaenoic acid rich oil lower fasting and postprandial plasma lipid levels. *Eur J Clin Nutr* 1996;50:765–771.

Åkesson C; Lindgren H; Pero RW; et al.; An extract of *Uncaria tomentosa* inhibiting cell division and NF-κB without inducing cell death. *J Int Immunopathology* (in press, 2003).

Åkesson C; Pero RW; Ivars F; C-Med-100, a hot water extract of *Uncaria tomentosa,* prolongs leukocyte survival *in vivo. Phytomed* 2003;10:25–33.

Albert CM; et al.; Blood levels of long-chain fatty acids and the risk of sudden death. *N Engl J Med* 2002;346:1113–1118.

Ames, BA; Micronutrients prevent cancer and delay aging. *Toxicol Lett* 1998; 102–103:5–18.

Ames, BA; Wakimoto P; Are vitamin and mineral deficiencies a major cancer risk? *Nat Rev Cancer* 2002;2:694–704.

Ames, BN; Elson-Schwab I; Silver EA; High-dose vitamin stimulates variant enzymes with decreased coenzyme binding affinity (increased Km): relevance of genetic disease and polymorphisms. *Am J Clin Nutr* 2002;75:616–658.

Bagchi M; et al.; Smokeless tobacco, oxidative stress, apoptosis and antioxidants in human oral keratinocytes. *Free Rad Biol Med* 1999;26:992–1000.

Barbiroli B; et al.; Lipoic (thioctic) acid increases brain energy availability and skeletal muscle performance as shown in vivo. ^{31}P-MRS in a patient with mitochondrial cytopathy. *J Neurol* 1995;2423:472–477.

Barclay L; Dietary omega-3 fatty acids may reduce risk of age-related macular degeneration. *Medscape,* May 14, 2003.

Barnes PJ; Karin M; Nuclear factor-κB—a pivotal transcription factor in chronic inflammatory diseases. *N Engl J Med* 1997;336:1066–1071.

Barringer TA; et al.; Effect of a multivitamin and mineral supplement on infection and quality of life. *Ann Intern Med* 2003; 138:365–371.

Beecher GR; Phytonutrients' role in metabolism: effects on resistance to degenerative processes. *Nutrition Rev* 1999;57:S3–S6.

Beg AA; Baltimore D; An essential role for NF-kappa B in preventing TNF-alpha-induced cell death. *Science* 1996;274:782–784.

Bianchi L; et al.; Carotenoids reduce the chromosol damage induced by bleomycin in human cultured lymphocytes. *Anticancer Res* 1993;13:1007–1010.

Bliznakov EG; Coenzyme Q$_{10}$, lipid-lowering drugs (statins) and cholesterol: a present day Pandora's box. *JANA* 2002;5:32–38.

Bliznakov EG; Wilkins DJ; Biochemical and clinical consequences of inhibiting coenzyme Q$_{10}$ biosynthesis by lipid-lowering HMG-CoA reductase inhibitors (statins): a critical overview. *Adv Therapy* 1998;15:218–228.

Bonnesen C; Eggleston IM; Hayes JD; Dietary indoles and isothiocyanates that are generated from cruciferous vegetables can both stimulate apoptosis and confer protection against DNA damage in human colon cell lines. *Cancer Res* 2001;61:6120–6130.

Borek C; Antioxidant health effects of aged garlic extract. *J Nutr* 2001;131: 1010S–1015S.

Borum PR; Carnitine. *Ann Rev Nutr* 1983;3:233–259.

Boyonoski AC; et al.; Niacin deficiency increases the sensitivity of rats to the short and long term effects of ethylnitrosourea treatment. *Mol Cell Biochem* 1999;193:83–87.

Boyonoski AC; et al.; Pharmacological intakes of niacin increase bone marrow poly(ADP-ribose) and the latency of ethylnitrosourea-induced carcinogenesis in rats. *J Nutr* 2002;132:115–120.

Bradlow HL; et al.; Multifunctional aspects of the action of indole-3-carbinole as an antitumor agent. *Ann NY Acad Sci* 1999;889:204–213.

Broquist HP; Carnitine. In Shils, ed., *Modern Nutrition in Health and Disease,* 8th ed. Philadelphia, PA: Lea & Febinger, 1994, pp 459–465.

Burge B; Mitochondria: the beleaguered powerhouse of the cell. *Healthline* 1999:10–11.

Cao LZ; Lin ZB; Regulatory effect of *Ganoderma lucidum* polysaccharides on cytotoxic T-lymphocytes induced by dendritic cells in vitor. *Acta Pharmacol Sin* 2003;24:312–326.

Ceda GP; et al.; Alpha-glycerylphosphorylcholine administration increases the GH responses to GHRH of young and elderly subjects. *Hormone Metab Res* 1991;24:119–121.

Cerhan JR; et al.; Antioxidant micronutrients and risk of rheumatoid arthritis in a cohort of older women. *Am J Epidemiol* 2003;157:345–354.

Chambers JC; et al.; Improved vascular endothelial function after oral B vitamins: an effect mediated through reduced concentrations of free plasma homocysteine. *Circulation* 2000;102:2479–2483.

Chandra RK; Effect of vitamin and trace-element supplementation on immune responses and infection in elderly subjects. *Lancet* 1992;340:1124–1127.

Chen DZ; et al.; Indole-3-carbinol and diindolylmethane induce apoptosis of human cervical cancer cells and in murine HPV16-transgenic preneoplastic cervical epithelium. *J Nutr* 2001;131:3294–3302.

Chew BP; et al.; A comparison of the anticancer activities of beta-carotene, canthaxanthin and astaxanthin in mice in vivo. *Anticancer Res* 1999;19: 1849–1853.

Clarke SD; et al.; Fatty acid regulation of gene expression. Its role in fuel partitioning and insulin resistance. *Ann NY Acad Sci* 1997;827:178–187.

Chopra RK; et al.; Relative bioavailability of coenzyme Q10 formulations in human subjects. *Int J Vit Nutr Res* 1997;68:109–113.

Collins, AR; et al.; Serum carotenoids and oxidative DNA damage in human lymphocytes. *Carcinogenesis* 1999;19:2159–2162.

Davi G; Ciabattoni G; Consoli A; In vivo formation of 8-isoprostaglandin F-2-alpha and platelet activation in diabetes mellitus. *Circulation* 1999;88:224–229.

Decker P; Briande JP; de Murcia G; Pero RW; et al.; Zinc is an essential cofactor for recognition of the DNA binding domain of poly(ADP-ribose) polymerase by antibodies in autoimmune rheumatic and bowel diseases. *Arthrit Rheum* 1998;41:918–926.

Devaraj S; Jialal I; Alpha-tocopherol supplementation decreases serum C-reactive protein and monocytes. Interleukin-6 levels in normal volunteers and type 2 diabetic patients. *Free Rad Biol Med* 2000;29:790–792.

Dillon SA; et al.; Dietary supplementation with aged garlic extract reduces plasma and urine concentrations of 8-iso-prostaglandin F_2 in smoking and nonsmoking men and women. *J Nutr* 2002;132:168–171.

Dulloo AG; et al.; Efficacy of a green tea extract rich in catechins, polyphenols, and caffeine in increasing 24-h energy expenditure and fat exidation in humans. *Am J Clin Nutr* 1999;70:1040–1045.

Earnest C; et al.; Efficacy of a complex multivitamin supplement. *Nutrition* 2002;18:738–742.

Engelhart MJ; et al.; Dietary intake of antioxidants and risk of Alzheimer disease. *JAMA* 2002;287:3223–3229.

Fernandez-Pol JA; Douglas MG; Molecular interactions of cancer and age. *Hematol Oncol Clin North Am* 2000;14:25–44.

Fleischauer AT; et al.; Dietary antioxidants, supplements, and risk of epithelial ovarian cancer. *Nutr Cancer* 2002;40:92–98.

Fletcher RH; Fairfield KM; Vitamins for chronic disease prevention. *JAMA* 2002;287:3127–3129.

Fujimura Y; et al.; Antiallergic tea catechins (-)-epigallocatechin-3-O-(3-O-methyl)-gallate, suppresses Fc epsilon RI expression in human basophilic KU812 cells. *J Agric Food Chem* 2002;50:5729–5734.

Fullerton SA; et al.; Induction of apoptosis in human prostatic cancer cells with B-glucan (maitake mushroom polysaccharide). *Mol Urol* 2000;4:7–13.

Ger E; Angelucci JA; Coleman P; Mushrooms: enjoying your medicine. *Delaware Med J* 1997;69:149–151.

Halpern GM; Miller AH; *Medicinal Mushrooms: Ancient Remedies for Modern Ailments.* New York: M. Evans and Co., 2002, pp 34–57.

Han DH; et al.; Relationship between estrogen receptor-binding and estrogenic activities of environmental estrogens and suppression by flavonoids. *Biosci Biotechnol Biochem* 2002;66:1479–1487.

Hano O; et al.; Coenzyme Q_{10} enhances cardiac functional and metabolic recovery and reduces Ca2+ overload during postischemic reperfusion. *Am J Physiol* 1994;266:H2174–2181.

Hecht SS; Chemoprevention of lung cancer by isothiocyanates. *Adv Exp Med Biol* 1996;401:1–11.

Hodges S; et al.; CoQ_{10}: Could it have a role in cancer management? *Biofactors* 1999;9:364–370.

Hu FB; et al.; Fish and omega-3 fatty acid intake and risk of coronary heart disease in women. *JAMA* 2002; 287:1815–1821.

Ide N; Lau BHS; Garlic compounds minimize intracellular oxidative stress and inhibit nuclear factor-κB activation. *J Nutr* 2001;131:1020S–1026S.

Jacques PF; The potential preventive effects of vitamins for cataract and age-related macular degeneration. *Int J Vitam Nutr Res* 1999;69:198–205.

Jain S; et al.; Effect of vitamin E supplementation on the hyperviscosity and hyper-coagulability of blood in diabetic patients. Dept. of Ped., Louisiana State Med. Center Study, 1998, pp 7–13 (unpublished).

Jenkinson A McE; et al.; The effect of increased intakes of polyunsaturated fatty acids and vitamin E on DNA damage in human lymphocytes. *FASEB J* 1999;3:2138–2142.

Jeong HJ; et al.; Inhibition of aromatase activity by flavonoids. *Arch Pharm Res* 1999; 22:309–312.

Jialal I; Fuller C; Huet B; The effect of alpha-tocopherol supplementation on LDL oxidation. *Arterioscler Thromb Vas Biol* 1995;15:190–198.

Judy WV; Stogsdill WW; Folkers K; Myocardial preservation by therapy with coenzyme Q_{10} during heart surgery. *Clin Investig* 1993;71:S155–S161.

Jump DB; Dietary polyunsaturated fatty acids and regulation of gene transcription. *Curr Opin Lipidol* 2002; 13:155–164.

Kawamori T; et al.; Chemoprevention of azoxymethane-induced colon carcinogenesis by dietary feeding of S-methyl methane thiosulfonate in male F344 rats. *Cancer Res* 1995;55:4053–4058.

Kendler BS; Nutritional strategies in cardiovascular disease control: an update on vitamins and conditionally essential nutrients. *Prog Cardiovasc Nurs* 1999;14:124–129.

Kiziltunc, et al.; Carnitine and antioxidant levels in patients with rheumatoid arthritis. *Scand J Rheumatol* 1998;27:441–445.

Knekt P; et al.; Flavonoid intake and risk of chronic diseases. *Am J Clin Nutr* 2002;76:560–568.

Krall EA; et al.; Calcium and vitamin D supplements reduce tooth loss in the elderly. *Am J Med* 2001;111:452–456.

Kwong LK; et al.; Effects of coenzyme Q_{10} administration on its tissue concentrations, mitochondrial oxidant generation, and oxidative stress in the rat. *Free Red Biol Med* 200;33:627–638.

Lau CS; Morley KD; Belch JJ; Effects of fish oil supplementation on non-steroidal anti-inflammatory drug requirements in patients with mild rheumatoid arthritis—a double-blind placebo controlled study. *Br J Rheumatol* 1993;32:982–989.

Lamm S; Pero RW; Persistent response to pneumococcal vaccine in individuals supplemented with a novel aqueous extract from *Uncaria tomentosa,* C-Med-100. *Phytomed* 2001;8:267–274.

Le HT; et al.; Plant-derived 3,3′-diindolylmethane is a strong androgen antagonist in human prostate cancer cells. *J Biol Chem* 2003;278:21136–21145.

Lipkin M; Early development of cancer chemoprevention clinical trials: studies of dietary calcium as a chemopreventive agent for human subjects. *Eur J Cancer Prev* 2002;11(suppl 2):S65–S70.

Liu L; Yeh YY; Inhibition of cholesterol biosynthesis by organosulfur compounds derived from garlic. *Lipids* 2000;35:197–203.

Liu J; et al.; Memory loss in old rats is associated with brain mitochondrial decay and RNA/DNA oxidation: partial reversal by feeding acetyl-L-carnitine and/or R-α-lipoic acid. *Proc Natl Acad Sci USA* 2002;99:2356–2361.

Lowe NM; et al.; Is there a potential therapeutic value of copper and zinc for osteoporosis? *Proc Nutr Soc* 2002;61:181–185.

Lyons NM; O'Brien NM; Modulatory effects of an algal extract containing astaxanthin on UVA-irradiated cells in culture. *J Dermatol Sci* 2002;30:73–84.

Matuoka K; Chen KY; Takenawa T; Rapid reversion of aging phenotypes by nicotinamide through possible modulation of histone acetylation. *Cell Mol Life Sci* 2001;58:2108–2116.

Maher TJ; L-Carnitine and coenzyme Q_{10}. *Natural Healing Track*, New Hope Institute of Natural Healing, March 2000.

Maher TJ; Alpha-lipoic acid and Co-Q10 in diabetes mellitus. *Natural Healing Track,* New Hope Institute of Natural Healing, July 2000.

Masaki KH; et al.; Association of vitamin E and C supplement use with cognitive function and dementia in elderly men. *Neurology* 2000;54:1265–1272.

Mennen LI; et al.; Homocysteine, cardiovascular disease risk factors, and habitual diet in the French Supplementation with Antioxidant Vitamins and Minerals Study. *Am J Clin Nutr* 2002;76:1279–1289.

Meydani, M; Vitamin E. *Lancet* 1995;345:170–175.

Meydani S; Meydani M; Blumberg J; Vitamin E supplementation and in vivo immune response in healthy elderly subjects. *J Am Med Assoc* 1997;277: 1380–1386.

Meyer F; et al.; Lower ischemic heart disease incidence and mortality among vitamin supplement users. *Canad J Cardiol* 1996;12:930–934.

Miles MV; et al.; Bioequivalence of coenzyme Q_{10} from over-the-counter supplements. *Nutr Res* 2002;33:919–929.

Morris MC; et al.; Vitamin E and cognitive decline in older persons. *Arch Neurol* 2002;60:292–293.

Mortensen SA; et al.; Dose-related decrease of serum coenzyme Q_{10} during treatment with HMG-CoA reductase inhibitors. *Molec Aspects Med* 1997;18:S137–144.

Nagamatsu M; et al.; Lipoic acid improves nerve blood flow, reduces oxidative stress, and improves distal nerve conduction in experimental diabetic neuropathy. *Diabetes Care* 1995;18:1160–1167.

Nakagawa S; Kasuga S; Matsuura H; Prevention of liver damage by aged garlic extract and its components in mice. *Phyto Res* 1988;1:1–4.

Nesaetnam K; Dorasamy S; Darbre PD; Tocotrienols inhibit growth of ZR-75-1 breast cancer cells. *Internat J Food Sci Nutr* 2000;51:95–103.

Packer L; Witt EH; Tritschler HJ; Alpha-lipoic acid as a biological antioxidant. *Free Rad Biol Med* 1995;19:227–250.

Panasenko; et al.; Interaction of peroxynitrite with carotenoids in human low density lipoproteins. *Arch Biochem Biophys* 2000;373:302–305.

Paolisso G; Amore A; Giugliano D; Pharmacologic doses of vitamin E improve insulin action in healthy subjects and non-insulin-dependent diabetic patients. *Am J Clin Nutr* 1993;57:650–656.

Paolisso G; et al.; Pharmacological doses of vitamin E and insulin action in elderly subjects. *Am J Clin Nutr* 1994;59:1291–1296.

Pero RW; Zimmerman M; The good news: natural DNA repair systems. In *Reverse Aging.* Chico, CA: Nutrition Solution Publications, 2002, pp 41–45.

Pero RW; et al.; Newly discovered anti-inflammatory properties of the benzamides and nicotinamides. *Mol Cell Biochem* 1999;193:119–125.

Pero RW; et al.; Formulation and clinical evaluation of combining DNA repair and immune enhancing nutritional supplements. *Phytomed* 2003; (in press).

Pero RW; Giampapa V; Vojdani A; Comparison of a broad spectrum anti-aging nutritional supplement with and without the addition of a DNA repair enhancing cat's claw extract. *J Anti-Aging Med* 2003;5:345–353.

Prasad K; et al.; Prevention of hypercholesterolemic atherosclerosis by garlic and antioxidant. *J Cardiovasc Pharmacol Ther* 1997;2(4):309–320.

Qureshi AA; et al.; Lowering of serum cholesterol in hypercholesterolemic humans by tocotrienols (Palmvee). *Am J Clin Nutr* 1991;53:1021S–1026S.

Ray B; Medicinal mushrooms. *Taste for Life,* May 2003, pp 35–38.

Reed J; Cranberry flavonoids, atherosclerosis and cardiovascular health. *Crit Rev Food Sci Nutr* 2002;42:301–316.

Regnstrom J; et al.; Inverse relation between the concentration of low-denisty lipoprotein vitamin E and severity of coronary artery disease. *Am J Clin Nutr* 1996;63:377–385.

Reid IR; et al.; Effects of calcium supplementation on serum lipid concentrations in normal older women: a randomized controlled trial. *Am J Med* 2002;112:343–347.

Ribaya-Mercado JD; et al.; Skin lycopene is destroyed preferentially over beta-carotene during ultraviolet irradiation in humans. *J Nutr* 1995;125: 1854–1859.

Rissanen TH; et al.; Serum lycopene concentrations and carotid atherosclerosis: the Kuopio Ischaemic Heart Disease Risk Factor Study. *Am J Clin Nutr* 2003;77:133–138.

Rosenberg Zand RS; et al.; Flavonoids can back PSA production by breast and prostate cancer cell lines. *Clin Chim Acta* 2002;317:17–26.

Russell IJ; et al.; Treatment of fibromyalgia syndrome with Super Malic: a randomized double blind, placebo controlled, crossover pilot study. *J Rheumatol* 1995;22:953–958.

Sandoval M; et al.; Cat's claw inhibits TNF alpha production and scavenges free radicals: role in cytoprotection. *Free Radic Biol Med* 2000;29:71–78.

Sandoval-Chacon M; et al.; Antiinflammatory actions of cat's claw: the role of NF-kappa B. *Ailment Pharmacol Ther* 1998;12:1279–1289.

Sato E; et al.; Antioxidants inhibit tumor necrosis factor-alpha mediated stimulation of interleukin-8, monocytes chemoattractant protein-1, and collagenase expression in cultured human synovial cells. *J Rheumatol* 1996;23: 432–438.

Scholmerich J; et al.; Bioavailability of zinc from zinc-histidine complexes. I. Comparison with zinc sulfate in healthy men. *Am J Clin Nutr* 2000;130:1378–1383.

Scholte HR; et al.; Primary carnitine deficiency. *J Clin Chem Clin Biochem* 1990;28:351–357.

Seth RK; Kharb S; Protective function of alpha-tocopherol against the process of cataractogenesis in humans. *Ann Nutr Metab* 1999;43:286–289.

Sheng Y; Pero RW; et al.; DNA repair enhancement by a combined supplement of carotenoids, nicotinamide and zinc. *Cancer Detect Prev* 1998;22:284–292.

Sheng Y; Bryngelsson C; Pero RW; Enhanced DNA repair, immune function and reduced toxicity of C-Med-100, a novel aqueous extract from *Uncaria tomentosa*. *J Ethnopharmacol* 2000;69:115–126.

Sheng Y; Li L; Hoomgren K; Pero RW; DNA repair enhancement of aqueous extracts of *Uncaria tomentosa* in a human volunteer study. *Phytomed* 2001;8:275–282.

Shils, ME; Olson, JA; Shike M; *Modern Nutrition in Health and Disease,* 8th ed. Philadelphia, PA: Lea & Febinger, 1994, pp 144–477.

Sies H; Stahl W; Sundquist AR; Antioxidant functions of vitamins. Vitamins E and C, beta-carotene, and other antioxidants. *Ann NY Acad Sci* 1002;669: 7–20.

Simon JA; Hudes ES; Serum ascorbic acid and other correlates of self-reported cataract among older Americans. *J Clin Epidemiol* 1999;52:1207–1211.

Snowdon DA; et al.; Serum folate and the severity of atrophy of the neocortex in Alzheimer disease: findings from the Nun Study. *Am J Clin Nutr* 2000; 71:993–998.

Stahl W; et al.; Carotenoids and carotenoids plus vitamin E protect against ultraviolet light–induced erythema in humans. *Am J Clin Nutr* 2000;71:795–798.

Stephenson PU; et al.; Modulation of cytochrome P4501A1 (CYP1A1) activity by ascorbingen in murine hepatome cells. *Biochem Pharmacol* 1999;58:1145–1153.

Stipanuk MH; *Biochemical and Physiological Aspects of Human Nutrition.* Philadelphia, PA: WB Saunders, 2000, pp 458–842.

Stoll AL; et al.; Choline ingestion increases the resonance of choline-containing compounds in human brain: an in vivo proton magnetic resonance study. *Biol Psychiat* 1995;37:170–174.

Streeper RS; et al.; Differential effects of lipoic acid stereoisomers on glucose metabolism in insulin-resistant skeletal muscle. *Am J Physiol* 1997;273: E185–E191.

Sreejayan N; Rao MN; Nitric oxide scavenging by curcuminoids. *J Pharm Pharmacol* 1997;49:105–107.

Sumioka I; et al.; Mechanisms of protection by S-allylmercaptocysteine against acetaminophen-induced liver injury in mice. *Japanese J Pharmacol* 1998;78: 199–207.

Sumioka K; Matsura T; Yamada K; Therapeutic effect of S-allylmercaptocysteine on acetaminophen-induced liver injury in mice. *Eur J Pharmacol* 2001;433:177–185.

Suzuki H; et al.; Cardiac performance and coenzyme Q_{10} in thyroid disorders. *Endocrinol Jpn* 1984;31:755–761.

Suzuki YJ; Packer L; et al.; Redox regulation of NF-κB DNA binding activity by dihydrolipoate. *Biochem Mol Biol Int* 1995;36:241–246.

Takayami Y; et al.; Vitamin E supplementation and endurance exercises: Are there benefits? *Sports Med* 2000;29:73–83.

Tang AM; et al.; Low serum vitamin B-12 concentrations are associated with faster human immunodeficiency virus type 1 (HIV-1) disease progression. *J Nutr* 1997;127:345–351.

Taylor A; et al.; Long-term intake of vitamins and carotenoids and odds of early age-related cortical and posterior subcapsular lens opacities. *Am J Clin Nutr* 2002;75:540–549.

Terry P; et al.; Dietary intake of folic acid and colorectal cancer risk in a cohort of women. *Int J Cancer* 2002;97:864–867.

Theriault A; et al.; Tocotrienol: a review of its therapeutic potential. *Clin Biochem* 1999;32:309–319.

Thomas PS; Heywood G; Effects of inhaled tumor necrosis factor alpha in subjects with mild asthma. *Thorax* 2002;57:774–778.

Uauy-Dagach R; Velenzuela A; Marine oils: the health benefits of n-3 fatty acids. *Nutr Rev* 1996;54:S102–108.

Valentine JS; Gralla EB; Delivering copper inside yeast and human cells. *Science* 1997;278:817–818.

van Tits L; et al.; Alpha-tocopherol supplementation decreases production of superoxide and cytokines by leukocytes ex vivo in both normolipidemic and hypertriglyceridemic individuals. *Am J Clin Nutr* 2000;71:458–464.

Vinson JA; Relative bioavailability of trace elements and vitamins found in commerical supplements. In *Nutrient Availability: Chemical and Biological Aspects.* Norwich, England: The Royal Society of Chemistry, 1989, pp 125–128.

Vinson JA; Bose P; Comparative bioavailability to humans of ascorbic acid alone or in a citrus extract. *Am J Clin Nutr* 1988;48:601–604.

Vinson JA; Howard TB; Inhibition of protein glycation and advanced glycation end products by ascorbic acid and other vitamins and nutrients. *J Nutr Biochem* 1996;7:659–663.

Vinson JA; Jang J; In vitro and in vivo lipoprotein antioxidant effect of a citrus extract and ascorbic acid on normal and hypercholesterolemic human subjects. *J Medicinal Food* 2001;4:187–192.

Wang CY; Mayo MW; Baldwin AS, Jr.: TNF- and cancer therapy-induced apoptosis: potentiation by inhibition of NF-κB *Science* 1996; 274:784–787.

Wang J; et al.; Overfeeding rapidly induces leptin and insulin resistance. *Diabetes* 2001;50:2786–2791.

Wargovich MJ; et al.; Aberrant crypts as a biomarker for colon cancer: evaluation of potential chemopreventive agents in the rat. *Cancer Epidemiol Biomarkers Prev* 1996;5:355–360.

Wartanowicz M; et al.; The effect of alpha-tocopherol and ascorbic acid on the serum peroxide level in elderly people. *Ann Nutr Metab* 1984;28:186–191.

Wasser SP; Review of medicinal mushrooms. *Advances HerbalGram* 2002;56: 29–33.

Webb D; Chromium connections: promising health roles surface at summit. *Environ Nutr* 2002;26:1, 4.

Yeh YY; Liu L; Cholesterol-lowering effect of garlic extracts and organosulfur compounds: human and animal studies. *J Nutr* 2001;131:989S–993S.

Yochum L; Folsom A; Kushi L; Intake of antioxidant vitamins and risk of death from stroke in postmenopausal women. *Am J Clin Nutr* 2000;72:476–483.

Yu W; et al.; Induction of apoptosis in human breast cancer cells by tocopherols and tocotrienols. *Nutr Cancer* 1999;33:26–32.

Zhang SM; et al.; Plasma folate, vitamin B6, vitamin B12, homocysteine, and risk of breast cancer. *J Natl Cancer Inst* 2003;95:373–380.

Ziamlanski S; et al.; The effect of two-year supplementation with ascorbic acid and alpha tocopherol on lipid, hematological and vitamin state in elderly women. *J Metabolism* 1986;13:7–14.

Ziegler D; Arnold GF; α-Lipoic acid in the treatment of diabetic peripheral and cardiac autonomic neuropathy. *Diabetes* 1997;46(suppl):S62–S66.

Zimmer G; et al.; Decrease of red cell membrane fluidity and SH groups due to hyperglycemic conditions is counteracted by α-lipoic acid. *Arch Biochem Biophys* 1995;342:85–92.

CHAPTER 7: STEP 5: MAKE OVER YOUR SKIN AND BODY

Akwa Y; et al.; Neurosteroids: biosynthesis, metabolism and function of pregnenolone and dehydroepiandrosterone in the brain. *J Steroid Biochem Mol Biol* 1991;40:71–81.

Ames BN; Micronutrients prevent cancer and delay aging. *Toxicol Letters* 1998;102–103:5–18.

Amri H; Armas I; Gonzalez N; The Bottom Line on HRT—Keynote Address. SOHO Expo, Orlando, Florida, December 12–15, 2002.

Andersson AM; Skakkebaek NE; Exposure to exogenous estrogens in food: possible impact on human development and health. *Eur J Endocrinol* 1999;140:477–485.

Ardies CM; Dees C; Xenoestrogens significantly enhance risk for breast cancer during growth and adolescence. *Med Hypotheses* 1998;50:457–464.

Arendt J; Biological rhythms: the science of chronobiology. *JR Coll Physicians Lond* 1998;32:27–35.

Armstrong SM; Redman JR; Melatonin: a chronobiotic with anti-aging properties? *Med Hypotheses* 1991;34:300–309.

Barrett-Connor E; Goodman-Gruen D; The epidemiology of DHEA-S and cardiovascular disease. *Ann NY Acad Sci* 1995;774:259–270.

Barrett-Connor E; et al.; Endogenous levels of dehydroepiandrosterone sulfate, but not other sex hormones, are associated with depressed mood in older women: the Rancho Bernardo Study. *J Am Geriatr Soc* 1999;47:685–691.

Beg AA; Baltimore D; An essential role for NF-kappa B in preventing TNF-alpha-induced cell death. *Science* 1996;274:782–784.

Bernton E; et al.; Adaptation to chronic stress in military trainees, adrenal androgens, testosterone, glucocorticoids, IFG-1, and immune function. *Ann NY Acad Sci* 1995;774:217–231.

Blazejova K; et al.; Sleep disorders and the 24-hour profile of melatonin and cortisol. *Sb Lek* 2000;101:347–351.

Buffington CK; et al.; Case report: amelioration of insulin resistance in diabetes with dehydroepiandrosterone. *Am J Med Sci* 1993;306:320–324.

Cagnacci A; Elliott JA; Yen SSC; Melatonin: a major regulator of the circadian rhythm of core temperature in humans. *J Clin Endocrin Metab* 1992;75: 447–452.

Colborn T; Endocrine Disrupters *(Environ Health Perspec)* 2002;110:335–348.

Cossette LJ; et al.; Combined effect of xenoestrogens and growth factors in two estrogen-responsive cell lines. *Endocrine* 2002;3:303–308.

Dahlitz M; et al.; Delayed sleep phase syndrome response to melatonin. *Lancet* 1991;337:1121–1124.

Dhooge W; et al.; Observations as to male fertility in the Flemish environment and health studies. *Folio Histochem Cytobiol* 2001;39 (suppl2):38–39.

Diamond EM; et al.; Effects of dehydroepiandrosterone sulfate and stress on hippocampal electrophysiological plasticity. *Ann NY Acad Sci* 1995;774: 304–307.

Eberlein-Konig B; Placzek M; Przybilia B; Protective effect against sunburn of combined systemic ascorbic acid (vitamin C) and D-alpha-tocopherol (vitamin E). *J Am Acad Dermatol* 1998;38;45–48.

Egerman RS; et al.; Dehydroepiandrosterone attenuates study-induced declines in insulin sensitivity in postmenopausal women. *Ann NY Acad Sci* 1995; 774:291–293.

Ferguson LR; Natural and human-made mutagens and carcinogens in the human diet. *Toxicology* 2002;181–182:79–82.

Fuchs J; Kern H; Modulation of UV-light induced skin inflammation by D-alpha-tocopherol and L-ascorbic acid: a clinical study using solar simulated radiation. *Free Radic Biol Med* 1998;25:1006–1012.

Fuchs J; Milbradt R; Antioxidant inhibition of skin inflammation induced by reactive oxidants: evaluation of the redox couple dihydrolipoate/lipoate. *Skin Pharmacol* 1994;7:278–284.

Guerrero JM; Reiter RJ; A brief survey of pineal gland-immune system interrelationships. *Endocr Res* 1992;18:91–113.

Guth L; Zhang A; Roberts E; Key role for pregnenolone in combination therapy that promotes recovery after spinal cord injury. *Proc Natl Acad Sci USA* 1994;91:12308–12312.

Herrington DM; et al.; Plasma dehydroepiandrosterone and dehydroepiandrosterone sulfate in patients undergoing diagnostic coronary angiography. *J Am Coll Cardiol* 1990;16:862–870.

Hornsby PJ; Biosynthesis of DHEA-S by the human adrenal cortex and its age-related decline. *Ann NY Acad Sci* 1995;774:29–46.

James SP; et al.; Melatonin administration in insomnia. *Neuropsychopharmacology* 1990;3:19–23.

Kaunitz AM; Use of combination hormone replacement therapy in light of recent data from the Women's Health Initiative. *Medscape Women's Health eJournal* 2002;7(4).

Kronenberg F; Fugh-Berman A; Complementary and alternative medicine for menopausal symptoms: a review of randomized, controlled trials. *Ann Intern Med* 2002;137:805–813.

Labrie F; et al.; DHEA and its transformation into androgens and estrogens in peripheral target tissues: intracrinology. *Front Neuroendocrinol* 2001;22: 185–212.

Lardy H; et al.; Induction of thermogenic enzymes by DHEA and its metabolites. *Ann NY Acad Sci* 1995;774:171–179.

Lee JR; *Natural Progesterone—The Multiple Roles of a Remarkable Hormone.* Sebastopol, CA: BLL Publications, 1993.

Leonetti HB; et al.; Transdermal progesterone cream for vasomotor symptoms and postmenopausal bone loss. *Gynecol* 1999;94:225–228.

Magnaghi V; et al.; Neuroactive steroids and peripheral myelin proteins. *Brain Res Brain Res Rev* 2001;37:360–371.

Majewska MD; Neuronal actions of dehydroepiandrosterone—possible roles in brain development, aging, memory, and affect. *Ann NY Acad Sci* 1995; 774:111–120.

Mani S; G protein-coupled receptor signaling in neuroendocrine systems: signaling mechanisms in progesterone-neurotransmitter interactions. *J Mol Endocrinol* 2002;30:127–137.

Maurizi CP; The therapeutic potential for tryptophan and melatonin: possible roles in depression, sleep, Alzheimer's disease and abnormal aging. *Med Hypotheses* 1990;31:233–242.

McDonald JD; et al.; Emissions from charbroiling and grilling of chicken and beef. *J Air Waste Manag Assoc* 2003;53:185–194.

Melchior CL; Ritzmann RF; Neurosteroids block the memory-impairing effects of ethanol in mice. *Pharmacol Biochem Behavior* 1996;53:51–56.

Milewich L; et al.; Pleotropic effects of dietary DHEA. *Ann NY Acad Sci* 1995; 774:149–170.

Moskowitz D; Changing views: the emergence of efficacy of natural hormones in the treatment of menopause. *JANA* 2003;3:36–44.

Murialdo G; et al.; Relationships between cortisol, dehydroepiandrosterone sulphate and insulin-like growth factor-I system in dementia. *J Endocrinol Invest* 2001;24:139–146.

Nestler JE; Regulation of human dehydroepiandrosterone metabolism by insulin. *Ann NY Acad Sci* 1995;774:73–81.

Norman AW; Litwack G; *Hormones,* 2nd ed. San Diego, CA: Academic Press, 1997.

Park SJ; Tokura H; Bright light exposure during the daytime affects circadian rhythms of urinary melatonin and salivary immunoglobulin A. *Chronbiol Int* 1999;16:359–371.

Pero RW; et al.; Newly discovered anti-inflammatory properties of the benzamides and nicotinamides. *Mol Cell Biochem* 1999;193:119–125.

Perricone NV; DiNardo JC; Photoprotective and anti-inflammatory effects of topical glycolic acid. *Dermatol Surg* 1996;22:435–437.

Pierpaoli W; Changxian Y; The involvement of pineal gland and melatonin in immunity and aging. *J Neuroimmunol* 1990;27:99–109.

Piscoya J; et al.; Efficacy and safety of freeze-dried cat's claw in osteoarthritis of the knee: mechanisms of action of the species *Uncaria guianensis. Inflamm Res* 2001;50:442–448.

Polleri A; et al.; Dementia: a neuroendocrine perspective. *J Endcrinol Invest* 2002;25:73–83.

Raloff, J; New concerns about phthalates. *Science News,* Sept 2, 2000; 158(10):152–154.

Raloff J; Girls may face risks from phthalates. *Science News,* Sept 9, 2000; 158(11):165.

Rebas E; Lachowicz A; Lachowicz L; Estradiol and pregnenolone sulfate could modulate PMA-stimulated and Ca2+/calmodulin-dependent synaptosomal membrane protein phosphorylation from rat brain in vivo. *Biochem Biophys Res Comm* 1995;207:606–612.

Reiter RJ; The aging pineal gland and its physiological consequences. *Bio Essays* 1992;14:169–175.

Reiter RJ; Oxidative processes and antioxidative defense mechanisms in the aging brain. *FASEB J* 1995;9:526–533.

Remesar X; et al.; Estrone in food: a factor influencing the development of obesity? *Eur J Nutr* 1999;38:247–253.

Rosano GM; et al.; Natural progesterone, but not medroxyprogesterone acetate, enhances the beneficial effect of estrogen on exercise-induced myocardial ischemia in postmenopausal women. *J Am Coll Cardiol* 2000;36:2154–2159.

Sandoval M; et al.; Cat's claw inhibits TNF alpha production and scavenges free radicals: role in cytoprotection. *Free Radic Biol Med* 2000;29:71–78.

Sandoval M; et al.; Antiinflammatory and antioxidant activities of cat's claw (*Uncaria tomentosa* and *Uncaria guianensis*) are independent of their alkaloid content. *Phytomedicine* 2002;9:325–327.

Sandoval-Chacon M; et al.; Antiinflammatory actions of cat's claw: the role of NF-kappa B. *Aliment Pharmacol Ther* 1998;12:1279–1289.

Sandyk R; Possible role of pineal, melatonin in the mechanisms of aging. *Int J Neuroscience* 1990;52:85–92.

Sandyk R; et al.; Is postmenopausal osteoporosis related to pineal gland functions? *Int J Neuroscience* 1992;62:215–225.

Schumacher M; et al.; Progesterone synthesis and myelin formation in peripheral nerves. *Brain Res Brain Res Rev* 2001;37:343–359.

Schwartz AG; Pashko LL; Mechanism of cancer preventive action of DHEA. *Ann NY Acad Sci* 1995;774:180–186.

Sheng Y; Pero RW; et al.; DNA repair enhancement by a combined supplement of carotenoids, nicotinamide, and zinc. *Cancer Detec Preven* 1998;22: 284–292.

Skakkebaek NE; Endocrine disrupters and testicular dysgenesis syndrome. *Horm Res* 2002;57 (suppl 2):43.

Smart RC; Crawford CL; Effect of ascorbic acid and its synthetic lipoplilic derivative ascorbyl palmitate on phorbol ester–induced skin-tumor promotion in mice. *Am J Clin Nutr* 1991;54 (suppl 6):1266S–1273S.

Stoffel-Wagner B; Neurosteroid metabolism in the human brain. *Eur J Endocrinol* 2002;145:669–679.

Tan RS; Pu SJ; The andropause and memory loss: Is there a link between androgen decline and dementia in the aging male? *Asian J Androl* 2001;3:169–174.

Tan DX; et al.; The pineal hormone melatonin inhibits DNA-adduct formation induced by the chemical carcinogen safrole in vivo. *Cancer Lett* 1993; 70:65–71.

Tebbe B; et al.; L-ascorbic acid inhibits UVA-induced lipid peroxidation and secretion of IL-1 alpha and IL-6 in cultured human keratinocytes *in vitro. J Invest Dermatol* 1997;108:302–306.

Teilmann G; et al.; Putative effects of endocrine disrupters on pubertal development in the human. *Best Pract Res Clin Endocrinol Metab* 2002;16:105–121.

Terzolo M; et al.; effects of long-term, low-dose, time-specified melatonin administration on endocrine and cardiovascular variables in adult men. *J Pineal Res* 1990;9:113–124.

Utiger RD; Testosterone "fix": youth or consequence? *Health News NEJM,* April, 2003;3.

Vermeulen A; Dehydroepiandrosterone sulfate and aging *Ann NY Acad Sci* 1995;774:121–142.

Wang CY; Mayo MW; Baldwin AS; TNF- and cancer therapy–induced apoptosis: potentiation by inhibition of NF-kappa B. *Science* 1996;274:784–787.

Weaver DR; et al.; Melatonin receptors in human hypothalamus and pituitary: implications for circadian and reproductive responses to melatonin. *J Clin Endocrinol Metabol* 1993;76:295–301.

Weisburger JH; Comments on the history and importance of aromatic and heterocyclic amines in public health. *Mutat Res* 2002;506–507:9–20.

Wolkowitz OM; et al.; Antidepressant and cognition-enhancing effects of DHEA in major depression *Ann NY Acad Sci* 1995;774:337–339.

Writing Group (WHI); Risks and benefits of estrogen plus progestin in healthy postmenopausal women: principal results from the Women's Health Initiative randomized controlled trial. *JAMA* 2002;288:321–333, 366–368.

Yamashita U; et al.; Effect of endocrine disrupters on immune responses *in vitro. J UOEH* 2002;24:1–10.

Appendix A: Anti-Aging Home Testing

Atherden SM; Development and application of a direct radioimmunoassay for aldosterone in saliva. *Steroids* 1985;46:845–855.

Banne AF; Amiri A; Pero RW; Reduced level of serum thiols in patients with a diagnosis of active disease. *J Anti-Aging Medicine* 2003 (in press).

Barrett-Connor E; Bioavailable testosterone and depressed mood in older men: the Rancho Bernado Study. *J Clin Endocrinol Metab* 1999;84:573–577.

Baruchel S; Wainberg MA; The role of oxidative stress in disease progression in individuals infected by the human immunodeficiency virus. *J Leuco Biol* 1992;52:111–114.

Beckman KB; Ames BN; The free radical theory of aging matures. *Psychol Rev* 1990;78:547–581.

Blazejova K; et al.; Sleep disorders and the 24-hour profile of melatonin and cortisol. *Sb Lek* 2000;101:347–351.

Block G; et al.; Factors associated with oxidative stress in human populations. *Am J Epidemiol* 2002;156:274–285.

Bohr V; et al.; Oxidative DNA damage processing and changes with aging. *Toxicol Lett* 1998;102–103:47–52.

Bolaji II; Sero-salivary progesterone correlation. *Int J Gynecol Obstet* 1994; 45:125–131.

Brenner DD; et al.; Biomarkers in styrene-exposed boat builders. *Mutation Res* 1991;261:225–236.

Cedard L; et al.; Progesterone and estradiol in saliva after in vitro fertilization and embryo transfer. *Fertility and Sterility* 1987;47:278–283.

Cortopassi GA; Wang E; There is substantial agreement among interspecies estimates of DNA repair activity. *Mech Aging Dev* 1996;13:211–218.

Dabbs JM; et al.; Salivary testosterone measurements: reliability across hours, days, and weeks. *Physiol Behav* 1990;48:83–86.

Dabbs JM; et al; Reliability of salivary testosterone measurements: a multicenter evaluation. *Clin Chem* 1995;41:1581.

Devaraj S; et al.; Divergence between LDL oxidative susceptibility and urinary F_2-isoprostanes as a measure of oxidative stress in type 2 diabetes. *Clin Chem* 2001;47:1974–1978.

Dworski R; et al.; Assessment of oxidant stress in allergic asthma by measurement of the major urinary metabolite of F2-isoprostane, 15-F2t-IsoP (8-iso-PGF2alpha). *Clin Exp Allergy* 2001;31:387–390.

Giubilei F; et al.; Altered circadian cortisol secretion in Alzheimer's disease: clinical and neuroradiological aspects. *J Neurosci Res* 2001;66:262–265.

Gotovtseva LP; Korotko GF; Salivary thyroid hormones in evaluation of the functional state of the hypophyseal-thyroid system. *Klin Lab Diagn* 2002; 7:9–11.

Grossi G; et al.; Associations between financial strain and the diurnal salivary cortisol secretion of long-term unemployed individuals. *Integr Physiol Behav Sci* 2001;36:205–219.

Grube K; Burkle A; Poly(ADP-ribose) polymerase activity in mononuclear leukocytes of 13 mammalian species correlates with species-specific life span. *Proc Natl Acad Sci* 1993;89:11759–11763.

Ishikawa M; et al.; The clinical usefulness of salivary progesterone measurement for the evaluation of the corpus luteum function. *Gynecol Obstet Invest* 2002;53:32–37.

Johnson SG; et al.; Direct assay for testosterone in saliva: relationship with a direct serum free testosterone assay *Clin Chem Acta* 1987;163:309–318.

Klentrou P; et al.; Effect of moderate exercise on salivary immunoglobulin A and infection risk in humans. *Eur J Appl Physiol* 2002;87:153–158.

Laudat MH; et al.; Salivary cortisol measurement: a practical approach to assess pituitary-adrenal function. *J Clin Endocrinol Metab* 1988;66:343–348.

Lawrence HP; Salivary markers of systemic disease: noninvasive diagnosis of disease and monitoring of general health. *J Can Dent Assoc* 2002;68:170–174.

Lemaire I; et al.; Stimulation of interleukin-1 and -6 production in alveolar macrophages by the neotropical liana, *Uncaria tomentosa* (Una de Gato). *J Ethnopharmacology* 1999;64:109–115.

Lewy AJ; The dim light melatonin onset, melatonin assays and biological rhythm researched in humans. *Biol Signals Recept* 1999;8:79–83.

Lieber MR; Warner-Lambert/Parke Davis Award Lecture: pathological and physiological double-strand breaks. Roles in cancer, aging, and the immune system. *Am J Pathol* 1998;153:1323–1332.

Lu Y; et al.; Salivary estradiol and progesterone levels in conception and nonconception cycles in women: evaluation of a new assay for salivary estradiol. *Fertil Steril* 1999;72:951–952.

Mandel ID; et al.; The diagnostic uses of saliva. *J Oral Pathol* 1990;19:119–125.

Mayer J; et al.; Biologic markers in ethylene oxide, exposed workers and controls. *Mutation Res* 1991;248:163–176.

Mejtek VA; High and low emotion events influence emotional stress perceptions and are associated with salivary cortisol response change in a consecutive stress paradigm. *Psychoneuroendocrinology* 2002;27:337–352.

Miletic ID; et al.; Salivary IgA secretion rate in young and elderly persons. *Physiol Behav* 1996;60:243–248.

Morgan CA; et al.; Hormone profiles in humans experiencing military survival training. *Biol Psychiatry* 2000;47:891–901.

Nagetgaal E; et al.; Correlation between concentrations of melatonin in saliva and serum in patients with delayed sleep phase syndrome. *Therapeut Drug Monitoring* 1998;20:181–183.

Obminski Z; Stupnicki R; Comparison of the testosterone-to-cortisol ratio values obtained from hormonal assays in saliva and serum. *J Sports Med Phys Fitness* 1997;37:50–55.

Obminski Z; et al.; Effect of acceleration stress on salivary cortisol and plasma cortisol and testosterone levels in cadet pilots. *J Physiol Pharmacol* 1997; 48:193–200.

Park SJ; Tokura H; Bright light exposure during the daytime affects circadian rhythms of urinary melatonin and salivary immunoglobulin A. *Chronobiol Int* 1999;16:359–371.

Pearson TA; et al.; Markers of inflammation and cardiovascular disease: application to clinical and public health practice: a statement for healthcare professionals from the Centers for Disease Control and Prevention and the American Heart Association. *Circulation* 2003;107:499–511.

Pero RW; Giampapa V; Oxidative stress and its effects on immunity and apoptosis—DNA repair as a primary molecular target for antiaging therapies (2001 position paper, unpublished).

Pero RW; Seidegard J; Miller DG; Development of biochemical markers sensitive to ecogenetic variation and their use in assessing risk from genotoxic exposures. *Prog Clin Biol Res* 1988;209B:225–235.

Pero RW; et al.; A reduced capacity for unscheduled DNA synthesis in lymphocytes from individuals exposed to propylene oxide and ethylene oxide. *Mutation Res* 1982;104:193–200.

Pero RW; et al.; Reduced capacity for DNA repair synthesis in patients with or genetically predisposed to colorectal cancer. *N Natl Cancer Inst* 1983;70: 867–875.

Pero RW; et al.; DNA repair synthesis as a marker of predisposition to colorectal cancer. *Prog Clin Biol Res* 1988;279:289–303.

Pero, RW; et al.; Oxidative stress induces DNA damage and inhibits the repair of DNA lesions induced by N-acetoxy-2-acetylaminofluorene in human peripheral mononuclear leukocytes. *Can Res* 1990;50:4619–4625.

Pero, RW; et al.; Oxidative stress, DNA repair, and cancer susceptibility. *Can Detec Prev* 1990; 14:555–561.

Pero RW; et al.; Hypochlorous acid/N-chloramines are naturally produced DNA repair inhibitors. *Carcinogenesis* 1996;17:13–18.

Pero RW; et al.; Serum thiols as a surrogate estimate of DNA repair correlates to mammalian life span. *J Antiaging Med* 2000;3:241–249.

Pero RW; et al.; Comparison of a broad spectrum anti-aging nutritional supplement with and without the addition of a DNA repair enhancing cat's claw extract. *J Antiaging Med* 2002;5(4):345–353.

Pero RW; et al.; Formulation and clinical evaluation of combining DNA repair and immune enhancing nutritional supplements (submitted *Phytomedicine*, 2003).

Peters JR; et al.; Salivary cortisol assays for assessing pituitary-adrenal reserve. *Clin Endocrinol* (Oxf) 1982;17:583–592.

Polleri A; et al.; Dementia: a neuroendocrine perspective. *J Endocrinol Invest* 2002;25:73–83.

Putz Z; et al.; Radioimmunoassay of thyroxin in saliva. *Clin Endocrinol* 1985;85:199–203.

differentiation   Process whereby a cell undergoes changes that convert it into a specialized cell.

disease genes   Genes that encode for abnormal proteins that cause disease.

DNA   Deoxyribonucleic acid, a double-stranded helix that carries the genetic code.

DNA adducts   Chemical changes in the DNA molecule that have not been specified by the four bases. DNA adducts are usually removed by excision repair.

DNA repair capacity   The ability of natural cellular processes to repair mistakes that occur in DNA.

DNA sequencing   Determining the order of nucleotides in a DNA molecule. It allows DNA to be studied in new ways. DNA sequencing is the primary goal of the Human Genome Project. *See also* **proteomics.**

DNA transcription   Copying of one strand of DNA onto a complementary copy of DNA or RNA. DNA transcription allows the expression of the genome.

doxorubicin (DXR)   A drug known to induce leucopenia, although it is designed to fight cancer.

electron acceptor   An atom or molecule that gains an electron from another atom or molecule and is thereby reduced. Redox reactions involve an electron acceptor and an electron donor. Oxygen accepts (steals) electrons from biomolecules to gain stability.

electron donor   An atom or molecule that gives an electron to another atom or molecule and is thereby oxidized. Fatty acids are one kind of molecule that donates electrons (not willingly) to oxygen. As a result, the fatty acid becomes oxidized and cannot function properly. Reactions such as these lead to oxidative stress.

electron transport   The movement of electrons along a chain of carrier molecules, going from higher-energy molecules to lower, and producing ATP in the process. During electron transport, some oxygen-free radicals are created.

encode   The process of giving exact genetic instructions for building proteins.

entropy   The degree of randomness in a system. Within the body, metabolism is normally well ordered. Oxidative stress induces entropy or disorder in metabolic processes.

enzyme   A protein that catalyzes a reaction between two or more atoms or molecules. Enzymes control all metabolic processes within the body.

excision repair   The most common kind of DNA repair. The damaged section of DNA is removed and replaced with the correct bases and sequence. The final step seals and strengthens the repaired area.

free radical   An atom or molecule with an unpaired electron. It lacks chemical stability, pulling electrons from stable molecules and setting off a chain reaction—rogue molecules that disrupt normal cell function by stealing electrons to gain molecular stability.

free radical theory of aging   Free radicals cause the progressive deterioration of biological systems over time. It's the predominant theory of how we age.

gap junction   The tiny connecting tubes or space between cells used to relay information between them.

gene sequencing   Mapping the specific order of nucleotide base pairs occurring in genes.

Quaggiotto P; Garag ML; Isoprostanes: indicators of oxidative stress in vivo and their biological activity. In TK Basu, ed., *Antioxidants and Human Health.* Australia: CAB International, 1999, pp 393–411.

Raff JL; et al.; Late-night salivary cortisol as a screening test for Cushing's syndrome. *J Clin Endocrinol Metab* 1998;83:2681–2686.

Rasmuson S; et al.; Increased glucocorticoid production and altered cortisol metabolism in women with mild to moderate Alzheimer's disease. *Biol Psychiatry* 2001;49:547–552.

Reiter RJ; Oxidative processes and antioxidative defense mechanisms in the aging brain. *FASEB* 1995;7:526–533.

Roberts LJ; Morrow JD; Measurement of F2-isoprostanes as an index of oxidative stress in vivo. *Free Rad Biol Med* 2000;28:505–513.

Roberts LJ; et al.; Novel eicosanoids. Isoprostanes and related compounds. *Methods Mol Biol* 1999;120:257–285.

Seidman SN; Testosterone deficiency and mood in aging men: pathogenic and therapeutic interactions. *World J Biol Psychiatry* 2003;4:14–20.

Swinkels LM; et al.; Low ratio of androstenedione to testosterone in plasma and saliva of hirsute women. *Clin Chem* 1992;38:1819–1823.

Szulc P; Delmas PD; Osteoporosis in the aged male. *Presse Med* 2002;31:1760–1769.

Tan RS; Pu SJ; The andropause and memory loss: Is there a link between androgen decline and dementia in the aging male? *Asian J Androl* 2001;3:169–174.

Thomas JA; Oxidative stress, oxidant defense, and dietary constituents. In M Shils, ed., *Modern Nutrition in Health and Disease.* Philadelphia: Lea & Febinger, 1994, pp 501–511.

Toniolo PG; et al.; A prospective study of endogenous estrogens and breast cancer in postmenopausal women *J Natl Cancer Inst* 1995;87:190–197.

Vienravi V; et al.; A direct radioimmunoassay for free progesterone in saliva. *J Med Assoc Thai* 1994;77:138–147.

Vittek J; et al.; Direct radioimmunoassay (RIA) of salivary testoterone: correlation with free and total serum testosterone. *Life Sci* 1985;37:711–716.

Voultsios A; et al.; Salivary melatonin as a circadian phase marker: validation and comparison to plasma melatonin. *J Biol Rhythms* 1997;12:457–466.

Vuorento T; et al.; Daily measurements of salivary progesterone reveal a high rate of anovulation in healthy students. *Scand J Clin Lab Invest* 1989;49:395–401.

Wang Z; et al.; Immunological characterization of urinary 8-epi-prostaglandin $F_{2\alpha}$ excretion in man. *J Pharmacol Environ Therapeutics* 1995;275:94–100.

Webley GE; Edwards R; Direct assay for progesterone in saliva: comparison with a direct serum assay. *Ann Clin Biochem* 1985;22:579–585.

Wong YF; et al.; Salivary estradiol and progesterone during the normal ovulatory menstrual cycle in Chinese women. *Gynecol Reprod Biol* 1990;34:129–135.

Worthman CM; et al.; Sensitive estradiol assay for monitoring ovarian function. *Clin Chem* 1990;36:1769–1773.

GLOSSARY

adenosine (A)   One of the four nucleotides that make up the chemistry of DNA and RNA. Adenosine is a purine. The other purine base is guanosine (G). Adenosine always pairs with thymidine (T).

adenosine triphosphate (ATP)   The energy-rich currency used by cells to drive metabolic reactions.

aging   The process of cellular breakdown primarily resulting from DNA damage.

alkaloid   Complex nitrogen-containing metabolite produced by plants that helps protect them against being eaten by herbivores. Alkaloids, caffeine being an example, are powerful pharmacological agents in humans.

allele   Humans carry two sets of chromosomes, one from each parent. An allele is one of the two (or more) forms of a particular gene.

anabolism/anabolic   Enzymatic reactions that build larger molecules from smaller ones.

anti-aging factors   Factors that delay or stop aging.

antibiotic   Substance that is toxic to microorganisms, thus limiting their growth.

antibody   Protein produced by B lymphocytes in response to a foreign molecule or invading organism.

antigen   Molecule that provokes the immune response to produce antibodies. An antigen can come from something outside the body such as undigested food particles, environmental contaminants, or pathogens.

antioxidants   Any of a large class of substances that neutralize free radicals before they cause damage.

apoptosis   Programmed cell death. Cells that have outlived their usefulness accept a signal to self-destruct, leaving younger, healthier cells to take up their functions. A protective process of cellular self-destruction.

autoantibody   Antibody that is formed in response to normal cellular constituents within the body. Autoantibodies are active in autoimmune disorders.

autoimmune   Immune attack against self.

B lymphocyte   A type of lymphocyte that differentiates into plasma cells that make antibodies. B cells also present antigens for destruction by cytotoxic T cells. Memory B cells recognize antigens that have been encountered before, a key function in the effectiveness of vaccination.

bacterial artificial chromosome (BAC)   A chromosome-like structure constructed by genetic engineering that carries genomic DNA to be cloned.

base   When combined with deoxyribose sugar and phosphate, this nitrogen-containing molecule is a building block of DNA called a nucleotide. Pyrimidine and purine are the nucleotides that make up the structure of DNA and RNA.

base pair   Two nucleotides (always a pyrimidine with a purine) that are paired and held together by a hydrogen bond.

basophil   A granulocytic white blood cell associated with allergic response. Basophils give rise to mast cells that release histamine during an allergic response in an effort to fight invading pathogens.

biological age   Your age according to your metabolic function as oppose[d] chronological age.

bradykinin   A neurohormone released during inflammation. Bradykin[in] important mediator of pain.

carboxy alkyl esters (CAEs)   The water-soluble actives in *Uncaria to*[mentosa] CAEs are a general chemical name indicating that all members contain functional group (i.e., carboxy) chemically bonded to an alcohol group.

carcinogen   An agent that causes cancer.

catabolism/catabolic   Enzyme-catalyzed reaction that breaks down comp[lex mol]ecules (fats, carbohydrates, and proteins) into energy-rich smaller m[olecules] such as ATP.

cell adhesion molecule   Protein on the surface of cells that mediates cell binding to form tissues and to transfer signals from one cell to another.

cell cycle   The orderly events in cellular reproduction. DNA replication is to this activity. Any defects in DNA can result in production of daught[er cells] (mutants) that cannot function properly.

cell-mediated immunity   Immune responses involving and direct[ed by] T lymphocytes.

centromere   Chromosomes contain a compact region known as a centr[omere] where sister chromatids (the two exact copies of each chromosome th[at are] formed after replication). This is the only place DNA strands are joined to[gether].

chromosomes   Tightly coiled strands of DNA and associated proteins that [make up] the genome.

chronological age   Your age in calendar years.

clone   Cells produced by repeated division of a single common cell or org[anism] that contains a single parent copy of DNA. This kind of reproduction is k[nown] as asexual because it does not involve two parents.

cloning   The process of generating exact copies of cells containing only one [set of] parent chromosomes. Cloning is asexual reproduction.

codon   A sequence of three nucleotides in a DNA or messenger RNA mol[ecule] that represents instructions for incorporation of a specific amino acid in a [pro]tein strand that is or should be built.

coenzyme   A small nonprotein molecule that attaches to an enzyme made of [pro]tein and is required for its activation. The coenzyme niacin (niacinamide) fo[rms] NAD and NADP, which are coenzymes for over 200 enzymatic reactions.

cosmeceutical   Agents that are active topically. These can be vitamins, mine[rals] semivitamins, or herbs.

C-reactive protein   A protein found in early stages of cardiovascular disease [and] some cancers.

cytokine   An extracellular signaling protein or peptide that acts as a local me[di]ator in cell-to-cell communication. Cytokines are important signaling prote[ins] in immune, nerve, and brain cell proliferation.

cytosine (C)   A pyrimidine base that always pairs with guanosine (G) in D[NA] strands.

cytotoxic T cell   A type of T lymphocyte that kills infected cells including canc[er] cells. They respond to antibody tags marking cells to be destroyed.

differentiated cells   Cells carrying the genetic code. They are fully functioning a[nd] highly specialized cells that carry out defined biochemical processes.

genetic control theory of aging   How we age is encoded in our genetic material.

genetic modifications   Small genetic changes that allow an organism to adapt and thus survive.

genome   The sequence of genes on DNA that spell out individual identity.

glycation   The cross-linking of proteins at the cellular and genetic levels caused by unregulated glucose levels, insulin surges, and insulin receptor insensitivity. Glycation directly affects gene expression and protein synthesis. Glycation of the immunoglobulin (Ig) molecule leads to altered function and may contribute to autoimmune reactions.

guanine (G)   A purine base that always pairs with cytosine (C) in DNA and uracil (G) in RNA.

histamine   A neurohormone released by mast cells during inflammation.

histones   Specialized structural proteins that suppress certain segments of DNA so that they are not transcribed. DNA is tightly coiled around histones.

in vitro   A biochemical process taking place in an isolated cell extract.

in vivo   A biochemical process taking place in a living organism.

junk DNA   Now called introns. Sections of DNA that do not contain genes but carry other important information for protein modification.

leucopenia   A condition in which numbers of white blood cells drop dramatically, leaving the immune system seriously impaired in fighting disease. Leucopenia is one result of chemotherapy.

lipids   Fatty oil-soluble substances. Biological membranes are made of lipids, a combination of phospholipids and long-chain polyunsaturated fatty acids.

macrophages   Large scavenging white blood cells.

mast cells   Widely distributed tissue cell that releases histamine during an inflammatory response.

messenger RNA (mRNA)   RNA molecule that specifies the amino acid sequence of a protein.

metabolic disorders   Those that involve a genetic error in sequencing an enzyme or enzymes involved in a specific metabolic pathway(s).

metabolism   The sum total of chemical reactions related to living. Metabolic processes are regulated by enzymes, which are proteins that catalyze changes in biomolecules driven by energy product or consumption.

methylation   The addition of a CH_3 (methyl group) that controls the masking of specific regions of DNA, in effect switching genes on or off. This alters how genetic messages are translated and modifies genetic expression.

mitogen   An agent that stimulates T-cells to divide. Phytohemagglutinin is one example.

molecular medicine   A branch of medicine that focuses on abnormalities in specific metabolic pathways involved in a disease.

NAD   Nicotine adenine dinucleotide, a coenzyme form of niacin (nicotinamide) that participates in redox reactions and produces energy.

NADP   Nicotine adenine dinucleotide phosphate, a niacin coenzyme that participates in biosynthetic pathways.

necrosis   Cells that die because they are injured or damaged in some way. Necrosis occurs from outside damage, whereas apoptosis occurs because of internal cellular signals.

neurohormone   A hormone that stimulates the brain and nerves.

neuropeptide   A peptide (small amino acid complex) secreted by neurons to transmit messages.

neurotransmitter   A small signaling molecule that relays chemical messages between the brain and nerve cells (neurons).

NF-κB   Nuclear factor kappa B is a nuclear transcription factor that regulates numerous genes encoding proteins that are important in apoptosis, inflammation, and cellular growth. Normally, NF-κB activates apoptosis to combat the free-radical hazards of oxidative stress.

nicotinamide   Vitamin B_3, also called niacin, nicotinic acid, a precursor of coenzymes NAD (nicotinamide adenine dinucleotide) and NADP.

nucleic acid   The base pairs that make up RNA and DNA.

nucleoside   A base, either a purine or pyrimidine that is chemically bonded to a sugar and phosphate.

nutraceuticals   Substances derived from food or herbs having pronounced pharmacological and medicinal effects.

oxidation   (specific definition) Loss of an electron by an atom or molecule, typically by addition of oxygen as in oxidation/reduction or redox reactions. Can also be the loss of a hydrogen atom or proton. (generalized definition) Free-radical damage produced at the intracellular and extracellular levels. Oxidation directly affects genetic structure and function and cell membrane and organelle function.

oxidative stress   The total body burden of molecules that have been damaged by oxygen-free radicals.

oxindole alkaloids   A group of six or more active components in *Uncaria* species sharing a similar organic nitrogen-containing structure.

phagocytes   White blood cells that engulf bacteria, viruses, or other foreign material.

phagocytosis   Process by which cells or other foreign material is eaten by white blood cells.

phospholipid   Lipid molecules used to construct biological membranes that act as biological soaps because they have both water-soluble and lipid-soluble ends.

polyunsaturated fatty acids (PUFAs)   Essential fatty acids that are elongated and desaturated (i.e., double bonds between carbon atoms) to form the long-chain PUFAs found in biomembranes.

product   The result of an enzymatically controlled chemical reaction.

protein   The major macromolecular constituent of cells, of which enzymes are one kind.

proteomics   The study of how proteins carry out DNA's genetic orders. Proteomics is the fastest-growing area to be generated from the Human Genome Project. The protein complement generated from DNA is vastly more complicated   than unraveling the genome because there are so many proteins, and defining what each does, plus how it works, is challenging to the new frontier of medical research.

purine   The larger of the two bases that make up DNA and RNA. Adenosine and guanine are purines. They only bond with pyrimidines.

pyrimidine   The smaller of the two bases that make up DNA and RNA. Cytosine and thymidine are pyrimidines. A pyrimidine and a purine bond to form a base pair.

reaction Any process that changes the arrangement of atoms or molecules.

recombinant DNA Any DNA molecule formed by joining DNA segments from different sources. Widely used in cloning of genes and genetic modification of organisms or foods such as soy or corn (GMOs).

reduction Adding an electron; the opposite of oxidation. Occurs in oxidation/reduction or redox reactions. Can be the loss of an oxygen molecule or the gain of a hydrogen atom.

replication Reproductive and exact duplication of DNA.

ribosome Cellular organelle where RNA synthesizes proteins.

RNA Ribonucleic acid; nucleic acid material that encodes for proteins. RNA receives its instructions by pairing with a single strand of DNA. Then it carries the genetic code into the ribosome, where it can be translated into the synthesis of new proteins. RNA contains uracil instead of cytosine.

saturated fatty acids Lipids with no double bonds in the carbon backbone. Saturated fats are solid at room temperature. Most animal fats are saturated.

sex chromosomes The X and Y chromosomes. A pair of X's occur in females and an X is paired with a Y in males.

signal transduction The initiation and carrying of messages between cells.

single nucleotide polymorphisms (SNPs) The smallest kind of genetic variations that allow a species to adapt to its environment. SNPs allow survival of a species and are unique to an individual.

stem cell research The study of stem cell reproduction and its applications.

stem cells Cells carrying the genetic code but that have not differentiated into specialized cells that perform a particular function.

sterols Natural products derived from triterpenes and having a steroid skeleton.

substrate An atom or molecule that is acted upon by an enzyme.

T cell Type of lymphocyte responsible for cell-mediated immunity. Subsets include helper, suppressor, cytotoxic, natural killer cells, and memory T cells. Also known by CD3, CD4 (helper), and CD8 (cytotoxic) because of the receptor proteins on their surfaces.

thymidine (T) One of the pyrimidine bases found in DNA and RNA. Thymidine always bonds with the purine base adenosine (A).

TNF alpha (α) A protein that is produced by white blood cells that initiates the killing of tumor cells. TNFα also promotes inflammation, activates NF-κB, and increases oxidative stress.

transcription factors Proteins that initiate the transfer of genetic information.

trans fats Fatty acids with an altered chemical configuration that may be a leading cause of cardiovascular disease. Trans fats are produced during the partial hydrogenation of unsaturated fatty acids.

triterpenes Hydrocarbons of biological origin having a 30-carbon skeleton. Quinovic acid glycosides, a class of active principles in *Uncaria* species, are an example.

uracil (U) A pyrimidine base that replaces cytosine in RNA.

zinc finger A structural motif found on many DNA-binding proteins that requires a zinc atom for activation.

INDEX

Quaggiotto P; Garag ML; Isoprostanes: indicators of oxidative stress in vivo and their biological activity. In TK Basu, ed., *Antioxidants and Human Health*. Australia: CAB International, 1999, pp 393–411.

Raff JL; et al.; Late-night salivary cortisol as a screening test for Cushing's syndrome. *J Clin Endocrinol Metab* 1998;83:2681–2686.

Rasmuson S; et al.; Increased glucocorticoid production and altered cortisol metabolism in women with mild to moderate Alzheimer's disease. *Biol Psychiatry* 2001;49:547–552.

Reiter RJ; Oxidative processes and antioxidative defense mechanisms in the aging brain. *FASEB* 1995;7:526–533.

Roberts LJ; Morrow JD; Measurement of F2-isoprostanes as an index of oxidative stress in vivo. *Free Rad Biol Med* 2000;28:505–513.

Roberts LJ; et al.; Novel eicosanoids. Isoprostanes and related compounds. *Methods Mol Biol* 1999;120:257–285.

Seidman SN; Testosterone deficiency and mood in aging men: pathogenic and therapeutic interactions. *World J Biol Psychiatry* 2003;4:14–20.

Swinkels LM; et al.; Low ratio of androstenedione to testosterone in plasma and saliva of hirsute women. *Clin Chem* 1992;38:1819–1823.

Szulc P; Delmas PD; Osteoporosis in the aged male. *Presse Med* 2002;31: 1760–1769.

Tan RS; Pu SJ; The andropause and memory loss: Is there a link between androgen decline and dementia in the aging male? *Asian J Androl* 2001;3:169–174.

Thomas JA; Oxidative stress, oxidant defense, and dietary constituents. In M Shils, ed., *Modern Nutrition in Health and Disease.* Philadelphia: Lea & Febinger, 1994, pp 501–511.

Toniolo PG; et al.; A prospective study of endogenous estrogens and breast cancer in postmenopausal women *J Natl Cancer Inst* 1995;87:190–197.

Vienravi V; et al.; A direct radioimmunoassay for free progesterone in saliva. *J Med Assoc Thai* 1994;77:138–147.

Vittek J; et al.; Direct radioimmunoassay (RIA) of salivary testoterone: correlation with free and total serum testosterone. *Life Sci* 1985;37:711–716.

Voultsios A; et al.; Salivary melatonin as a circadian phase marker: validation and comparison to plasma melatonin. *J Biol Rhythms* 1997;12:457–466.

Vuorento T; et al.; Daily measurements of salivary progesterone reveal a high rate of anovulation in healthy students. *Scand J Clin Lab Invest* 1989;49: 395–401.

Wang Z; et al.; Immunological characterization of urinary 8-epi-prostaglandin $F_{2\alpha}$ excretion in man. *J Pharmacol Environ Therapeutics* 1995;275:94–100.

Webley GE; Edwards R; Direct assay for progesterone in saliva: comparison with a direct serum assay. *Ann Clin Biochem* 1985;22:579–585.

Wong YF; et al.; Salivary estradiol and progesterone during the normal ovulatory menstrual cycle in Chinese women. *Gynecol Reprod Biol* 1990;34:129–135.

Worthman CM; et al.; Sensitive estradiol assay for monitoring ovarian function. *Clin Chem* 1990;36:1769–1773.

GLOSSARY

adenosine (A) One of the four nucleotides that make up the chemistry of DNA and RNA. Adenosine is a purine. The other purine base is guanosine (G). Adenosine always pairs with thymidine (T).

adenosine triphosphate (ATP) The energy-rich currency used by cells to drive metabolic reactions.

aging The process of cellular breakdown primarily resulting from DNA damage.

alkaloid Complex nitrogen-containing metabolite produced by plants that helps protect them against being eaten by herbivores. Alkaloids, caffeine being an example, are powerful pharmacological agents in humans.

allele Humans carry two sets of chromosomes, one from each parent. An allele is one of the two (or more) forms of a particular gene.

anabolism/anabolic Enzymatic reactions that build larger molecules from smaller ones.

anti-aging factors Factors that delay or stop aging.

antibiotic Substance that is toxic to microorganisms, thus limiting their growth.

antibody Protein produced by B lymphocytes in response to a foreign molecule or invading organism.

antigen Molecule that provokes the immune response to produce antibodies. An antigen can come from something outside the body such as undigested food particles, environmental contaminants, or pathogens.

antioxidants Any of a large class of substances that neutralize free radicals before they cause damage.

apoptosis Programmed cell death. Cells that have outlived their usefulness accept a signal to self-destruct, leaving younger, healthier cells to take up their functions. A protective process of cellular self-destruction.

autoantibody Antibody that is formed in response to normal cellular constituents within the body. Autoantibodies are active in autoimmune disorders.

autoimmune Immune attack against self.

B lymphocyte A type of lymphocyte that differentiates into plasma cells that make antibodies. B cells also present antigens for destruction by cytotoxic T cells. Memory B cells recognize antigens that have been encountered before, a key function in the effectiveness of vaccination.

bacterial artificial chromosome (BAC) A chromosome-like structure constructed by genetic engineering that carries genomic DNA to be cloned.

base When combined with deoxyribose sugar and phosphate, this nitrogen-containing molecule is a building block of DNA called a nucleotide. Pyrimidine and purine are the nucleotides that make up the structure of DNA and RNA.

base pair Two nucleotides (always a pyrimidine with a purine) that are paired and held together by a hydrogen bond.

basophil A granulocytic white blood cell associated with allergic response. Basophils give rise to mast cells that release histamine during an allergic response in an effort to fight invading pathogens.

biological age Your age according to your metabolic function as opposed to your chronological age.

bradykinin A neurohormone released during inflammation. Bradykinin is an important mediator of pain.

carboxy alkyl esters (CAEs) The water-soluble actives in *Uncaria tomentosa*. CAEs are a general chemical name indicating that all members contain an acid functional group (i.e., carboxy) chemically bonded to an alcohol group.

carcinogen An agent that causes cancer.

catabolism/catabolic Enzyme-catalyzed reaction that breaks down complex molecules (fats, carbohydrates, and proteins) into energy-rich smaller molecules such as ATP.

cell adhesion molecule Protein on the surface of cells that mediates cell-to-cell binding to form tissues and to transfer signals from one cell to another.

cell cycle The orderly events in cellular reproduction. DNA replication is central to this activity. Any defects in DNA can result in production of daughter cells (mutants) that cannot function properly.

cell-mediated immunity Immune responses involving and directed by T lymphocytes.

centromere Chromosomes contain a compact region known as a centromere, where sister chromatids (the two exact copies of each chromosome that are formed after replication). This is the only place DNA strands are joined together.

chromosomes Tightly coiled strands of DNA and associated proteins that carry the genome.

chronological age Your age in calendar years.

clone Cells produced by repeated division of a single common cell or organism that contains a single parent copy of DNA. This kind of reproduction is known as asexual because it does not involve two parents.

cloning The process of generating exact copies of cells containing only one set of parent chromosomes. Cloning is asexual reproduction.

codon A sequence of three nucleotides in a DNA or messenger RNA molecule that represents instructions for incorporation of a specific amino acid in a protein strand that is or should be built.

coenzyme A small nonprotein molecule that attaches to an enzyme made of protein and is required for its activation. The coenzyme niacin (niacinamide) forms NAD and NADP, which are coenzymes for over 200 enzymatic reactions.

cosmeceutical Agents that are active topically. These can be vitamins, minerals, semivitamins, or herbs.

C-reactive protein A protein found in early stages of cardiovascular disease and some cancers.

cytokine An extracellular signaling protein or peptide that acts as a local mediator in cell-to-cell communication. Cytokines are important signaling proteins in immune, nerve, and brain cell proliferation.

cytosine (C) A pyrimidine base that always pairs with guanosine (G) in DNA strands.

cytotoxic T cell A type of T lymphocyte that kills infected cells including cancer cells. They respond to antibody tags marking cells to be destroyed.

differentiated cells Cells carrying the genetic code. They are fully functioning and highly specialized cells that carry out defined biochemical processes.

differentiation   Process whereby a cell undergoes changes that convert it into a specialized cell.

disease genes   Genes that encode for abnormal proteins that cause disease.

DNA   Deoxyribonucleic acid, a double-stranded helix that carries the genetic code.

DNA adducts   Chemical changes in the DNA molecule that have not been specified by the four bases. DNA adducts are usually removed by excision repair.

DNA repair capacity   The ability of natural cellular processes to repair mistakes that occur in DNA.

DNA sequencing   Determining the order of nucleotides in a DNA molecule. It allows DNA to be studied in new ways. DNA sequencing is the primary goal of the Human Genome Project. *See also* **proteomics.**

DNA transcription   Copying of one strand of DNA onto a complementary copy of DNA or RNA. DNA transcription allows the expression of the genome.

doxorubicin (DXR)   A drug known to induce leucopenia, although it is designed to fight cancer.

electron acceptor   An atom or molecule that gains an electron from another atom or molecule and is thereby reduced. Redox reactions involve an electron acceptor and an electron donor. Oxygen accepts (steals) electrons from biomolecules to gain stability.

electron donor   An atom or molecule that gives an electron to another atom or molecule and is thereby oxidized. Fatty acids are one kind of molecule that donates electrons (not willingly) to oxygen. As a result, the fatty acid becomes oxidized and cannot function properly. Reactions such as these lead to oxidative stress.

electron transport   The movement of electrons along a chain of carrier molecules, going from higher-energy molecules to lower, and producing ATP in the process. During electron transport, some oxygen-free radicals are created.

encode   The process of giving exact genetic instructions for building proteins.

entropy   The degree of randomness in a system. Within the body, metabolism is normally well ordered. Oxidative stress induces entropy or disorder in metabolic processes.

enzyme   A protein that catalyzes a reaction between two or more atoms or molecules. Enzymes control all metabolic processes within the body.

excision repair   The most common kind of DNA repair. The damaged section of DNA is removed and replaced with the correct bases and sequence. The final step seals and strengthens the repaired area.

free radical   An atom or molecule with an unpaired electron. It lacks chemical stability, pulling electrons from stable molecules and setting off a chain reaction—rogue molecules that disrupt normal cell function by stealing electrons to gain molecular stability.

free radical theory of aging   Free radicals cause the progressive deterioration of biological systems over time. It's the predominant theory of how we age.

gap junction   The tiny connecting tubes or space between cells used to relay information between them.

gene sequencing   Mapping the specific order of nucleotide base pairs occurring in genes.

genetic control theory of aging   How we age is encoded in our genetic material.

genetic modifications   Small genetic changes that allow an organism to adapt and thus survive.

genome   The sequence of genes on DNA that spell out individual identity.

glycation   The cross-linking of proteins at the cellular and genetic levels caused by unregulated glucose levels, insulin surges, and insulin receptor insensitivity. Glycation directly affects gene expression and protein synthesis. Glycation of the immunoglobulin (Ig) molecule leads to altered function and may contribute to autoimmune reactions.

guanine (G)   A purine base that always pairs with cytosine (C) in DNA and uracil (G) in RNA.

histamine   A neurohormone released by mast cells during inflammation.

histones   Specialized structural proteins that suppress certain segments of DNA so that they are not transcribed. DNA is tightly coiled around histones.

in vitro   A biochemical process taking place in an isolated cell extract.

in vivo   A biochemical process taking place in a living organism.

junk DNA   Now called introns. Sections of DNA that do not contain genes but carry other important information for protein modification.

leucopenia   A condition in which numbers of white blood cells drop dramatically, leaving the immune system seriously impaired in fighting disease. Leucopenia is one result of chemotherapy.

lipids   Fatty oil-soluble substances. Biological membranes are made of lipids, a combination of phospholipids and long-chain polyunsaturated fatty acids.

macrophages   Large scavenging white blood cells.

mast cells   Widely distributed tissue cell that releases histamine during an inflammatory response.

messenger RNA (mRNA)   RNA molecule that specifies the amino acid sequence of a protein.

metabolic disorders   Those that involve a genetic error in sequencing an enzyme or enzymes involved in a specific metabolic pathway(s).

metabolism   The sum total of chemical reactions related to living. Metabolic processes are regulated by enzymes, which are proteins that catalyze changes in biomolecules driven by energy product or consumption.

methylation   The addition of a CH_3 (methyl group) that controls the masking of specific regions of DNA, in effect switching genes on or off. This alters how genetic messages are translated and modifies genetic expression.

mitogen   An agent that stimulates T-cells to divide. Phytohemagglutinin is one example.

molecular medicine   A branch of medicine that focuses on abnormalities in specific metabolic pathways involved in a disease.

NAD   Nicotine adenine dinucleotide, a coenzyme form of niacin (nicotinamide) that participates in redox reactions and produces energy.

NADP   Nicotine adenine dinucleotide phosphate, a niacin coenzyme that participates in biosynthetic pathways.

necrosis   Cells that die because they are injured or damaged in some way. Necrosis occurs from outside damage, whereas apoptosis occurs because of internal cellular signals.

neurohormone   A hormone that stimulates the brain and nerves.

neuropeptide   A peptide (small amino acid complex) secreted by neurons to transmit messages.

neurotransmitter   A small signaling molecule that relays chemical messages between the brain and nerve cells (neurons).

NF-κB   Nuclear factor kappa B is a nuclear transcription factor that regulates numerous genes encoding proteins that are important in apoptosis, inflammation, and cellular growth. Normally, NF-κB activates apoptosis to combat the free-radical hazards of oxidative stress.

nicotinamide   Vitamin B_3, also called niacin, nicotinic acid, a precursor of coenzymes NAD (nicotinamide adenine dinucleotide) and NADP.

nucleic acid   The base pairs that make up RNA and DNA.

nucleoside   A base, either a purine or pyrimidine that is chemically bonded to a sugar and phosphate.

nutraceuticals   Substances derived from food or herbs having pronounced pharmacological and medicinal effects.

oxidation   (specific definition) Loss of an electron by an atom or molecule, typically by addition of oxygen as in oxidation/reduction or redox reactions. Can also be the loss of a hydrogen atom or proton. (generalized definition) Free-radical damage produced at the intracellular and extracellular levels. Oxidation directly affects genetic structure and function and cell membrane and organelle function.

oxidative stress   The total body burden of molecules that have been damaged by oxygen-free radicals.

oxindole alkaloids   A group of six or more active components in *Uncaria* species sharing a similar organic nitrogen-containing structure.

phagocytes   White blood cells that engulf bacteria, viruses, or other foreign material.

phagocytosis   Process by which cells or other foreign material is eaten by white blood cells.

phospholipid   Lipid molecules used to construct biological membranes that act as biological soaps because they have both water-soluble and lipid-soluble ends.

polyunsaturated fatty acids (PUFAs)   Essential fatty acids that are elongated and desaturated (i.e., double bonds between carbon atoms) to form the long-chain PUFAs found in biomembranes.

product   The result of an enzymatically controlled chemical reaction.

protein   The major macromolecular constituent of cells, of which enzymes are one kind.

proteomics   The study of how proteins carry out DNA's genetic orders. Proteomics is the fastest-growing area to be generated from the Human Genome Project. The protein complement generated from DNA is vastly more complicated   than unraveling the genome because there are so many proteins, and defining what each does, plus how it works, is challenging to the new frontier of medical research.

purine   The larger of the two bases that make up DNA and RNA. Adenosine and guanine are purines. They only bond with pyrimidines.

pyrimidine   The smaller of the two bases that make up DNA and RNA. Cytosine and thymidine are pyrimidines. A pyrimidine and a purine bond to form a base pair.

reaction Any process that changes the arrangement of atoms or molecules.

recombinant DNA Any DNA molecule formed by joining DNA segments from different sources. Widely used in cloning of genes and genetic modification of organisms or foods such as soy or corn (GMOs).

reduction Adding an electron; the opposite of oxidation. Occurs in oxidation/reduction or redox reactions. Can be the loss of an oxygen molecule or the gain of a hydrogen atom.

replication Reproductive and exact duplication of DNA.

ribosome Cellular organelle where RNA synthesizes proteins.

RNA Ribonucleic acid; nucleic acid material that encodes for proteins. RNA receives its instructions by pairing with a single strand of DNA. Then it carries the genetic code into the ribosome, where it can be translated into the synthesis of new proteins. RNA contains uracil instead of cytosine.

saturated fatty acids Lipids with no double bonds in the carbon backbone. Saturated fats are solid at room temperature. Most animal fats are saturated.

sex chromosomes The X and Y chromosomes. A pair of X's occur in females and an X is paired with a Y in males.

signal transduction The initiation and carrying of messages between cells.

single nucleotide polymorphisms (SNPs) The smallest kind of genetic variations that allow a species to adapt to its environment. SNPs allow survival of a species and are unique to an individual.

stem cell research The study of stem cell reproduction and its applications.

stem cells Cells carrying the genetic code but that have not differentiated into specialized cells that perform a particular function.

sterols Natural products derived from triterpenes and having a steroid skeleton.

substrate An atom or molecule that is acted upon by an enzyme.

T cell Type of lymphocyte responsible for cell-mediated immunity. Subsets include helper, suppressor, cytotoxic, natural killer cells, and memory T cells. Also known by CD3, CD4 (helper), and CD8 (cytotoxic) because of the receptor proteins on their surfaces.

thymidine (T) One of the pyrimidine bases found in DNA and RNA. Thymidine always bonds with the purine base adenosine (A).

TNF alpha (α) A protein that is produced by white blood cells that initiates the killing of tumor cells. TNFα also promotes inflammation, activates NF-κB, and increases oxidative stress.

transcription factors Proteins that initiate the transfer of genetic information.

trans fats Fatty acids with an altered chemical configuration that may be a leading cause of cardiovascular disease. Trans fats are produced during the partial hydrogenation of unsaturated fatty acids.

triterpenes Hydrocarbons of biological origin having a 30-carbon skeleton. Quinovic acid glycosides, a class of active principles in *Uncaria* species, are an example.

uracil (U) A pyrimidine base that replaces cytosine in RNA.

zinc finger A structural motif found on many DNA-binding proteins that requires a zinc atom for activation.

INDEX